Why Eat Like Jesus Ate?

How to get healthy and prevent
disease by following the
nutritional principles in the Bible.

by

Lorrie Medford, C.N.

LDN Publishing
P.O. Box 54007
Tulsa, Oklahoma 74155

WHY EAT LIKE JESUS ATE?
How to get healthy and prevent
disease by following the
nutritional principles in the Bible.

ISBN #0-9676419-7-7
Copyright © 2004 Lorrie Medford, C.N.
LDN Publishing
P. O. Box 54007
Tulsa, OK 74155

Unless otherwise noted, all Scripture references are taken from *The King James Version.* (See Bibles Referenced at the end of this book.) Scripture quotations are italicized.

Library of Congress Cataloging-in-Publishing Data

Medford, Lorrie

      Why Eat Like Jesus Ate?
      Lorrie Medford, C.N.
      International Standard Book Number: 0-9676419-7-7
      1. Nutrition 2. Health 3. Self Improvement I.Title

NOTE: This book is not intended to take the place of medical advice. Readers are advised to consult their doctor or other qualified healthcare professional regarding treatment of their medical conditions. The names of my clients have been changed. Any similarity to a real person is purely coincidental.

Printed in the United States of America

10 9 8 7 6 5 4 3 2 1 First U. S. Edition

(To order copies of this book, refer to the back pages of this book.)

Contents

Beloved, I wish above all things that thou mayest prosper and be in health, even as thy soul prospereth.

3 John 2

Foreword

I've known Lorrie Medford for several years. Along with my three daughters and lots of friends, we have had many opportunities to glean from Lorrie's expertise. The thing I appreciate most about her work is a balance of body, soul and spirit.

God wants us whole, and according to 3 John 2, it's in every area of our lives. As Lorrie has dedicated her life to teaching us how to follow biblical principles of wellness and wholeness, I've had much to learn, and appreciate her willingness to take the time to walk me through the process.

I personally thank God for her benefit to my family. It's very refreshing to find someone who believes the Word of God, and who wants to help God's people maintain abundant health.

Lindsay Roberts
Oral Roberts University
Tulsa, Oklahoma

Therefore thou shalt keep the commandments of the Lord thy God, to walk in His ways, and to fear Him.

For the Lord thy God bringeth thee into a good land, a land of brooks of water, of fountains and depths that spring out of valleys and hills;

A land of wheat, and barley, and vines, and fig trees, and pomegranates; a land of oil olive, and honey;

A land wherein thou shalt eat bread without scarceness, thou shalt not lack any thing in it; a land whose stones are iron, and out of whose hills thou mayest dig brass.

When thou hast eaten and art full, then thou shalt bless the Lord thy God for the good land which he hath given thee.

Deuteronomy 8:7-11

Acknowledgements

Many thanks to Lindsay Roberts, who so graciously wrote the foreword to this book, and who herself has a passion for both the Bible and nutrition. Her daily television show, "Make Your Day Count," has been a wonderful "pulpit" for teaching the Body of Christ about health and nutrition.

Many thanks to my precious clients, many of whom are Christians, who have encouraged me over the past several years to publish this book.

I'm grateful to several "health minded" friends. Brenda Richards, who read this book nearly three years ago said that she thought it was one of the most important books I have written. Thanks also to Bible/nutrition minded friends, Julie Wideman, Wendy Tatro and Linda Pereff who all recently read my book thoroughly. I appreciate your time, friendship and support in producing this book.

Nutrition is so vital to God that He has raised up many Christian health professionals to teach God's Word on health. Special thanks go to several Christian health professionals and authors whom I have quoted in this book: Dr. Reginald Cherry, Dr. Don Colbert, and Dr. Patrick Quillin.

I'm always grateful to my own staff, Anne Spears and Carolyn Clark who manage to juggle client orders and appointments, while supporting the production of my books. You both helped me so much on this book; I don't know what I would have done without you! You went above and beyond your job descriptions! Thanks for all of the time you spent helping me look up references and quotes, researching both nutrition and Bible verses. But even more important, thanks for all of your support, prayer and encouragement. You are both precious and I'm so grateful to have you as my assistants and friends.

Thanks to our sweet friend, Evie North, for doing the bookcover and numerous other projects. Your gift is truly from God!

Many thanks to Lori Oller, for your great edit. Your talent, focus, compassion and feedback are always so welcome and appreciated.

All of our gifts, talents and desires are given to us from God. So finally, I thank God with all of my heart. It was such a blessing to get to study and reflect on the Word of God as well as nutrition for this project. What a powerful combination!

God has done a mighty work in my life and continues to do so in the life of Believers. After I received Jesus as my Lord and Savior in 1985, my life and my health changed tremendously. I felt peace in my heart for the first time in my life. It doesn't mean that I don't have trials and circumstances to deal with. It just means that now I have God to help guide my life in a new way.

If you have never received Jesus as your Lord and Savior, you can receive Him right now by praying this prayer.

"Lord Jesus, I ask you to forgive me of all my sins. I believe that you died on the cross for me. According to Romans 10:9 and 10, if I confess with my mouth and believe in my heart that God raised Jesus from the dead, I shall be saved. I repent for my sins and receive Jesus as my Lord and Savior."

If you have prayed that prayer, I recommend that you find a Bible believing church and listen to anointed teachers. One of my favorites is Joyce Meyer, who ministers on TV and radio around the world. Her web site is www.joycemeyer.org.

What a great and mighty God we serve!

About the Author

Author and motivational speaker, Lorrie Medford has a B.A. in Communications and is a licensed Certified Nutritionist from The American Health Science University. She also holds certification as a personal trainer from The International Sports Science Association (ISSA). She is a member of the Oklahoma Speaker's Association and she also serves on the Advisory Board for Standard Process, Inc.

In addition to writing this book, she has also written *Why Can't I Stay Motivated?*, *Why Can't I Lose Weight?*, *Why Can't I Lose Weight Cookbook*, *Why Do I Need Whole-Food Supplements?*, *Why Am I So Grumpy, Dopey and Sleepy?*, *Why Do I Feel So Lousy?* and *Why Am I So Wacky?*

A health researcher and journalist, Lorrie has studied nutrition, whole-foods cooking, herbs, health, fitness, and motivation for more than 20 years. Lorrie taught her weight-loss class at a local junior college and through her own business for more than 10 years, and has taught natural foods cooking classes in Spokane, Washington and Tulsa, Oklahoma for 5 years.

She shares her knowledge in her seminars, and through her thriving nutritional consultation practice, *Life Design Nutrition,* in Tulsa, Oklahoma.

Lorrie has a rich history of community involvement teaching nutrition and is a sought-after speaker for civic groups, churches, hospitals, and wellness organizations. She is uniquely qualified to write about health and fitness. Lorrie knows what it's like to be a *cranky calorie counter* obsessed with foods, dieting, and striving to be thin. After struggling with her weight for many years, Lorrie lost more than 35 pounds and has kept it off for more than nineteen years.

Great multitudes followed Him (Jesus),
and He healed them all.
Matthew 12:15

Did Jesus Get Sick?

Do you think Jesus ever told His disciples, "Hey, guys, let's feed the 5,000 people tomorrow—I really don't feel up to it right now. I've got a cold, a sore throat, and a headache that won't quit!"

No! Jesus, who was our greatest example of life and health, was never sick. He wasn't overweight. He didn't have aches and pains. He didn't have arthritis or heart disease.

What Are You Praying For?

Listen to the prayer requests at church—are they for saving the lost? Not always. Often, they're for Christians who are sick. They are overweight. They have aches and pains. They have arthritis and heart disease.

Christians should be the healthiest people in the world because God wrote the first book on health.

If we didn't know better, we might think that God created us and said, "Here you go. Now fend for yourselves and go find food to eat. Hope you figure it all out!"

But no—the One who designed our bodies, also designed our foods, and gave us guidelines for health.

May I Have a Christian Pizza?

Look at the average shopping cart of a Christian and you won't see much difference from anyone else's cart: pizza, soda, French fries, and ice cream (otherwise known as the Basic Four Food Groups). "And why shouldn't we eat the same foods?" you might ask. "After all, there may be

Christian bookstores, but as of yet, there are no Christian supermarkets!"

Health and God Go Together

God created our bodies for specific foods that He knew would keep us healthy and give us long life. Today, biochemists and nutritionists are confirming these truths in their laboratories, continually validating ancient scriptures.

But Christians tend to read right over the Bible references to food. Even pastors probably preach about everything but nutrition. After all, there is no First and Second Book of Nutrition in the Bible!

By not studying God's Word regarding health, we actually are perishing for lack of knowledge (Hosea 4:6). And we are accidentally disobeying God's laws concerning health.

As a practicing Certified Nutritionist, I meet with wonderful Christians every day who have health problems. Most of them are living Godly lives, but they come to my office with symptoms of nutritional or hormonal imbalance.

For a Christian, not understanding God's Word on health is like getting a car and never reading the manual and then wondering why the car doesn't run. If they would have only read the owner's manual—the Word of God—they would know what God intended for us.

By not following His laws, we end up following the ideas of food manufacturers and advertisers. Now we're just as sick and tired as the world. This is not what God intended! He wants us to be an example of health for the world. God wanted us to be full of His Word, yes, but also full of His energy and health!

My pastor, Eastman Curtis, wrote in his foreword to my weight-loss book, "If we are going to accomplish the vision and destiny God has for us, a healthy body, clear mind and an abundance of physical energy are essential."

The Bible deals with **every** part of our lives. Second Timothy 3:16 says that the Bible is inspired by God for doctrine, reproof, correction and instruction in righteousness. I believe this means telling us how to live, including what to eat and how to eat, especially through the example of Jesus.

In *The Message Bible,* Hebrews 12:2 tells us to *keep your eyes on Jesus who both began and finished this race we're in. Study how He did it.*

Jesus was God, but He also lived in a physical body. We can learn about nutrition and health when we study how Jesus ate and the diet of the people who lived in Bible times.

How To Use This Book

There are four parts to this book.

· *Part One: God Designed You Well*

Chapter 1 tells how we were designed for health and long life. *Chapter 2* tells why as a nation, we are sick and getting sicker, instead of getting healthier.

· *Part Two*: *Is Processed Food Better Than God's Food?*

Chapter 3 begins with a look at various food guides, including the Food Guide Pyramid and Mediterranean Pyramid. *Chapters 4* to *7* look at various food processing methods and what they have done to our bodies and our health.

· *Part Three: God Cares About What You Eat*

Chapters 8 and *9* give revelation about God's Dietary Law in the Old and New Testaments. *Chapter 10* shows us how all of His foods are designed for healing and how to incorporate Bible foods in your daily menus.

· *Part Four: Pick Up Your Shield of Faith!*

Chapters 11, 12 and *13* give us a spiritual perspective on God's part and our part, self control, dealing with temptation and fasting.

Let's begin by looking at how wonderfully God made us.

PART ONE

God Designed You Well!

You created my inmost being. My frame was not hidden from you when I was made in the secret place.

When I was woven together in the depths of the earth, your eyes saw my unformed body.

Psalm 139:14-16 (NIV)

Chapter One

Your Wonderful Body

Can you imagine what life would be like if we were in charge of managing the life-sustaining functions of our bodies? How well would we do?

Don't Forget to Breathe!

Possibly, we could tell by our results: Poor Janice! She forgot to tell her blood to circulate to her left arm, and she only remembered after it became numb. And Ken... Breathe, Ken, Breathe! Or poor John—it look's like he forgot to tell his hair to grow on his head today.

Absurd, isn't it? Keeping our own bodies together would be a full-time job! Who needs this on top of everything else we have to do daily? Thank God that all of these functions are automatic.

For years I took my body, and how it worked, for granted. And then I took an in-depth anatomy and physiology class. We studied the incredibly intricate functions and organization of all of the body systems, and how they all work together, keeping our lungs breathing, our foods digesting, and our hearts beating. Whew! An amazing, great God designed us in an incredible way!

Your Incredible Body

In Psalm 139:13-14 of *The Living Bible (TLB)* the translators wrote, *You made all the delicate, inner parts of my body and knit them together in my mother's womb.* They called our bodies "wonderfully complex" and "marvelous."

Here is a small example of how amazing your body is. In your layers of skin, there are "sensors." Some are for pressure, some are for temperature. Your vascular system is designed in such a way to allow you to breathe in oxygen, have it go through your heart, then through all of your capillaries throughout your body and then back through your heart and out of your mouth—all simultaneously!

Your body contains trillions of cells which are continually replacing themselves. Sixty thousand miles of blood vessels pump blood throughout your body. Your heart beats about once every second, or 100,000 times a day. Your liver handles over 500 functions, producing over 1,000 different enzymes to handle all of the chemical conversions in your body. It is pretty amazing. You probably aren't even conscious of any of these actions.

Your Body Knows How To Heal

Not only is your body incredibly well organized, it's also self-regenerating and self-healing. Parts of your body are renewed every week, some are rebuilt every year. For example, every month, the outer layer of your skin is replaced. Every two months, most of the cells in your heart are rebuilt. Every year, the cells in your bones are replaced.

You can witness God's healing power every day. When your son or daughter falls down and scrapes their knee, immediately the body starts to repair itself. We don't have to "do" anything to make it heal, although we can help by cleaning the wound.

We're Supposed To Be Healthy!

Every part of our digestion and metabolism was designed to keep us active for a full, long life. Our bodies are incredibly designed with self-healing processes, provided we take care of them.

And how do you explain those people who seem healthy, but aren't? Perhaps they exercised regularly, didn't drink alcohol, and didn't smoke. Yet one day they "mysteriously" got sick or even died of heart disease or cancer. How could this happen to such wonderful Christian people?

It's easy to blame the cause of sickness on factors such as our age, genes or even the devil. But when it comes to our body and health, these aren't the most important factors. That's because God established certain laws **in our bodies** that dictate our health. If we break these laws of nature, we have to pay—sooner or later. You already have experienced this. Haven't you ever gone on a sugar binge and woken up the next day with a headache or other symptoms? Or, if you miss several meals, doesn't your body tell you about it?

What are these laws? Your cells are designed perfectly to take in food for your organs and tissues, and to release waste. Sounds easy, right? So what can go wrong? What if the food doesn't get into the cell, or the cell can't eliminate waste? This is an example of what happens when we go against God's natural laws or design of our bodies.

Think of the way we put a key into a lock; if it's the right key, it fits in naturally. Have you ever tried to jam the wrong key into a lock? This could break the key. Imagine trying to "jam" food into your cells that wasn't designed to go in there. This can damage the cell wall. If you get enough damage, then there are consequences. We call this disease.

Your body tries to make new cells every day. Without proper nutrition it can't make healthy cells. So the next generation of cells is weaker.

For centuries, clinical studies have proved that the better we eat, the healthier we are. But when were you taught about your body's natural healing processes and the foods that are healing? Because of lack of education, we often take better care of our cars than we do our bodies. You wouldn't, for example, put cheap fuel in your car. But few people realize the impact of foods on their health, or even know what were the "good" foods that Jesus ate.

God Wants You Well

There are so many, many references regarding how God designed us for health that entire books have been written about it, but here is one verse from *The King James Version*:

Exodus 15:26:

> *If thou wilt diligently hearken to the voice of the Lord thy God, and wilt do that which is right in his sight, and wilt give ear to his commandments, and keep all his statutes, I will put none of these diseases upon thee, which I have brought upon the Egyptians; for I am the Lord that healeth thee.*

Notice that in this reference, there is our part (listen to the Lord, do right, listen to His commandments), and God's part (health and healing). If God planned healing for us, we must be falling short of His design by knowingly or unknowingly not following His laws.

Live Long and Prosper

God promises more than just health; He promises a long life. Psalm 91:16 says, *With long life will I satisfy him, and shew* (show) *him my salvation.*

We shouldn't start falling apart just because we are getting older. God designed us to live a long life, and a good quality of life. He didn't want us to live to be 40 or 50 and start losing our hair, gaining weight, and getting tired!

Anyone who has read the Old Testament knows there were some extremely long-lived people, ranging from 600 to 900 years old! In the exciting field of nutrition, there is a great deal of literature about life extension and life enhancement, especially within the last ten years. Hundreds of articles have been written about the wonderful benefits of many foods for longevity.

Clinical research by one longevity author, Dr. Roy Walford, in his book, *Beyond the 120-Year Diet,* suggests that it is clearly possible for man to live as long as 120 years, as mentioned in Genesis 6:3.[1]

1 Cor. 6:19-20 says that we are the temple of the Holy Spirit. I believe this verse encourages us to glorify God with good health in our wonderful bodies. But are we?

Let's go to the next chapter which helps us understand why we are sick and getting sicker.

Chapter Two

Why Are We Sick and Getting Sicker?

Let's imagine some Aliens came to visit us from Mars. We quickly get to know them, and decide we should have dinner together. We run down to the supermarket and buy enough pizza and cokes to feed the neighborhood. Wanting to be polite, the friendly Martians put aside their "Green Grub" and eat pizza and drink soda. Pretty soon all of the Aliens are throwing up all the pizza and soda!

You could probably understand why all of the Aliens got sick. They had their own "Green Grub" designed perfectly for their Martian bodies. They weren't designed to eat pizza and drink soda.

So we shouldn't be too surprised if we get sick when we eat foods that were not designed for our bodies. People are always asking me, "Does nutrition really matter that much? "

In the Bible, it mattered to a young man named Daniel. Daniel would have really been successful by today's standards since he was attractive, intelligent and strong. And he was a terrific example of healthy living.

Better Than Fast Food

A short summary of the Book of Daniel is that the king requested the best young people to serve in his palace—youth "without blemish, well favored in appearance and skillful in all wisdom." And he had a royal meal plan for these youth: "rich and dainty" food, complete with wine. This plan probably included the rich meats and sweet desserts of the day, food only the affluent could afford. But Daniel decided not to eat the king's food. He requested a simple, healthy diet of vegetables and water to drink. At the end of ten days, he and his friends were looking better and healthier than all the youth who ate the king's rich food (Daniel 1:3-21 *AMP*).

We, like Daniel, should outshine others in our skill, intelligence and labor. We should be the healthiest people around. But we're not.

In his book, *What Would Jesus Eat?*, Dr. Don Colbert wrote that in 1901 the United States was the healthiest nation in the world among one hundred nations studied. By 1920, we dropped to second place. By 1950, we were in third place, and by 1981, we dropped to ninety-fifth place.[2] In spite of the trillions of dollars we spend on "health" care, America is one of the sickest nations in the world.

Look at These Statistics

Today, the top three killers include cancer, heart disease and diabetes. These diseases are not caused by bacteria, but a combination of malnutrition and toxic conditions. The medical care costs for Americans with chronic diseases such as these totals more than $400 billion annually.

The National Center for Health Statistics gave the ten leading causes of death in the U.S. for the year 2000: Here are some of their findings.[3]

1. **About 709,894 people died from heart disease.** Heart disease is still the nation's number one cause of death.

2. **About 551,833 people died from cancer.**

The World Health Organization (WHO) estimates deaths from cancer will double over the next 20 years.[4]

3. **About 68,662 people died from diabetes.** In 2000, diabetes was the nation's sixth cause of death, associated with excessive calories and obesity. In addition, there are about eight million undiagnosed diabetics.

Is Food Important?

Food is so important to God that He tells us what to eat in the first chapter of the first book of the Bible (Genesis 1:29), at the end of the Bible (Rev. 22:2) and throughout the Bible. God gave Adam and Eve the first "dietary guidelines."

In Genesis 2:16-17, God commanded Adam and Eve to eat certain foods and not to eat other foods. We are the temple, or the physical container of the Holy Spirit, and God wants us to know His Word regarding nutrition.

First Cor. 3:17 says, *If any man defile the temple of God, him shall God destroy.*

God designed a perfect diet for us. If we follow it, we will have health, energy, strength and a long life. If we don't follow it, or even accidentally eat the wrong foods, it will cause us death.

But not knowing how to eat from a Biblical perspective, we are influenced by the world. The media and food industry teach us what to like. We thought it didn't matter. And now we are paying the price.

Let's Go Back in Time

Okay, in the beginning, most people died from being eaten by a wild animal, such as a dinosaur or some other unfortunate circumstance. But I understand other than that, they were pretty healthy!

Let's go back fifty years ago, when the big killer diseases were smallpox, diphtheria and tuberculosis. These illnesses were caused by infectious bacteria. Unsanitary living conditions caused these epidemics. Next came processed, chemicalized foods which caused malnutrition. Did you know there was no reported incidence of heart disease until the early 1900s? Just one hundred years ago, only 3% of Americans died from cancer.

Sickness doesn't happen without a cause. There is a verse that says, *The curse causeless shall not come* (Proverbs 26:2).

Before the 1900s people didn't go to doctors for every pain and sniffle. In fact back then, there were more "natural doctors" who prescribed home remedies as well as drugs.

After the advent of food processing, which caused multiple vitamin and mineral deficiencies, people became encouraged to go to doctors for help. Drug companies came on the scene, and today there are drugs or surgery for everything. Doctors are trained in surgical procedures, not preventive medicine. They are schooled in medical emergencies and trauma. They are not taught to look for root causes such as nutritional deficiencies. Drugs are prescribed which often take away the symptoms, but don't get to the cause of the problem. Drugs can't heal, you but foods can.

Here are two verses that show that God's design for physical healing was with food:

And the fruit thereof shall be for meat, and the leaf therof for medicine (Ezekiel 47:12)

And the leaves of the tree were for the healing of the nations (Revelation 22:2)

Here are some common examples of various nutritional deficiencies in our American diet which cause disease:

Vitamin A deficiency causes dry scaly skin, acne, dry, dull hair, night blindness and increases susceptibility to illness.

Vitamin B deficiency causes depression, weak immune function, irritability or anxiety, and stress.

Vitamin C deficiency causes bruising, bleeding gums, joint pain, chronic fatigue, and nosebleeds.

Vitamin D deficiency causes soft teeth and/or tooth decay, thinning of bones, cracked teeth, and lower back pain.

Vitamin E deficiency causes liver spots, infertility, swollen legs, blood clots, heart disease, and cold hands and feet.

Calcium deficiency causes joint pain, leg cramps, back pain, and soft teeth.

Magnesium deficiency can cause irregular heartbeat, constipation, muscle cramps and muscular weakness.

Chromium deficiency can cause blood sugar problems, chronic fatigue, poor muscle tone and sugar cravings.

Medical drugs were created by man to relieve physical symptoms. While it's good that there are drugs to relieve symptoms, drugs are not God's best for us. Quite often, our symptoms start out as some type of nutritional imbalance which could be handled with whole-food nutritional supplements, dietary changes and even whole-food herbal supplements—at half the cost of the medications.

Today we know that many diseases can be prevented with proper nutrition and lifestyle! For the past twenty years, a tremendous amount of research has proved that malnutrition is a **major** contributor to disease and that proper nutrition can help **prevent** disease.

Here's how Elmer Josephson puts it in *God's Key to Health and Happiness:*[5]

> As it is not in God's plan to keep you alive without eating, so it is not in God's plan to keep you well without eating right! If you do not eat food you will die; if you do not eat good food you will not have good health.

A Drug for Every Symptom

Americans spend billions of dollars a year on drugs. Nutritionist Carol Simontacchi in her book, *Crazy Makers*, reports that the drug Prozac ranks fifth in the top ten pharmaceuticals, and over $7 billion is spent yearly on anti-depressants.[6] Yet I've helped people eliminate depression with various nutritional supplements.

I'm not opposed to doctors, appropriate drugs and surgery. **But drugs were not God's best for our healing.** God warned us against the deception of drugs. In the following verse, the word sorceries comes from the Greek word, "Pharmakia" which means "drugs."

For by thy sorceries were all nations deceived.

Revelation 18:23

All drugs are foreign to the body and toxic. If you have ever seen a Physician's Desk Reference (PDR), you would have seen that every drug has a side effect, even common over-the-counter medications.

People accept drugs prescribed by a doctor without any thought and assume they are safe. But every drug has serious side effects and thousands of people are affected by drugs. In an article in the *Washington Post* entitled, "Correctly Prescribed Drugs Take Heavy Toll," Rick Weiss wrote:[7]

> More than 2 million Americans become seriously ill every year because of toxic reactions to correctly prescribed medicines taken properly, and 106,000 die from those reactions, a new study concludes. That surprisingly high number makes drug side effects at least the sixth...most common cause of death in this country.

Drug companies spend billions of dollars on television advertisements, and they downplay the side effects. It would be better if commercials dramatized the side effects as well as the benefits. For example, you see a handsome man taking medicine for his allergies. Then you see him running to the nearest bathroom when the diarrhea hits!

I like how nutritionist Dr. Patrick Quillin puts it in his book, *Healing Secrets From the Bible.*[8]

> I have worked with many patients who were defying all of God's laws: eating poor food, smoking, not getting any exercise, living a stressful life, not praying, and not dealing with their body loaded with toxins which fasting would help. Without a thought for changing this semi-suicidal lifestyle, the doctor puts the patient on an endless array of prescription drugs, which all have dastardly side effects, until the patient eventually develops a really serious disease, like cancer. **We arrogantly assume that drugs can reverse the abuse caused by decades of poor nutrition and toxic burden. We are not respecting God's law of nature.**

What about synthetic female hormones which have been prescribed for 30 years? The first study published was from the huge Women's Health Initiative and included 16,000 women. This study which was supposed to be for 8 years, had to be stopped three years early when results showed that women using Premarin and Provera had a 29 percent higher risk of breast cancer, a 26 percent higher risk of heart disease, and a 41 percent higher risk of stroke. My female clients who have been on these drugs reported side effects of depression, irritability and weight gain. One client was named Janice.

When Janice came to see me she was taking several antidepressants. She was so "wacky" that she told me at the end of the appointment, that if I hadn't given her some answers, she was going to commit suicide that day! The drugs made her worse. But she didn't have a drug deficiency; she had numerous nutrient deficiencies. She's still doing well with the nutritional supplements I recommended.

In *Dr. Wright's Guide to Healing With Nutrition,* he writes:

> A congressional report concludes that only 10 to 20 percent of present-day "scientific" medical procedures has been shown to be of benefit by controlled clinical trails. One possible interpretation of this congressional document is that 80 to 90 percent of modern scientific medicine has no better scientific proof behind it than snake oil![9]

If drugs worked, we should be the healthiest country in the world and we should have overcome cancer, heart disease, and diabetes by now!

In the traditional Chinese medical system, doctors were paid to keep you well; if you got sick, they didn't get paid! They spent hundreds of years studying the human body in relationship to herbs and natural forms of healing. Their results are often quite amazing.

In view of the high cost of health insurance, we have it backwards, don't you think? It's one thing to spend hundreds of thousands of dollars on medicine and surgery, but another thing to not get the results or even feel that much better.

A fascinating book which discusses drugs and natural alternatives is called, *Amazing Medicines The Drug Companies Don't Want You to Discover* by Kugler and Revel.

Why are Christians sick? We have multiple nutritional deficiencies. Rather than look to foods, herbs and prayer, we look to doctors and drugs. Other drugs are prescribed to offset the bad effects of the first drug. God has a better plan for us!

Let's now look at man's dietary standards.

PART TWO

Is Processed Food Better Than God's Food?

Why spend your money on foodstuffs
that don't give you any strength?
Why pay for groceries that don't do you any good?
Isaiah 55:2 (TLB)

Chapter Three

The Many Dietary Food Guides for Americans

Can you imagine Adam and Eve in the garden looking for Twinkies or Ding Dongs? Besides, we read in Genesis that what they really liked was apples!

But have you ever wondered how we got to where we are? How were things in the beginning? When was the shift made from apples to McNuggets? Did Eve ever cook or order out in the Garden?

There's a history to everything, even food. In this chapter let's look at the different "dietary" standards.

Most of my younger clients are surprised to learn that the Food Guide Pyramid hasn't always been the standard that the government promoted in our country. There have been several government-recommended dietary standards throughout the years. First, there was the "Basic Twelve," which was changed to a "Basic Seven," which eventually changed to the popular, "Basic Four," and finally the Food Guide Pyramid, which contains six food groups and is currently under revision.

The American Way

I've been passionate about healthy eating since my early twenties, when I first began researching for my nutrition classes. That was when I found an article by Nathaniel Altman entitled, "Nutrition and Watergate: The Story of the Four Food Groups."[10] Each dietary change the government made became worse, omitting more food groups until it was only the "Basic Four." The "Basic Four" automatically became a national guideline for both Christians and non-Christians. There was never a scientific study to support these old Food Groups. There was never any report that said, "It has been proven that by drinking more milk and eating more meat, you will live longer and be healthier." We all accepted the grouping as the "American" way of life. Even Christians.

Here is what each dietary group included:

Basic Twelve (1930s)	Basic Seven (1940s)	Basic Four (1956)
1. Milk, dairy prod.	1. Milk, milk products	1. Milk
2. Potatoes, sweet potatoes	2. Tomatoes & fruits	2. Meat
3. Dry peas, beans, nuts	3. Leafy greens	3. Vegetables & fruits
4. Tomatoes & citrus fruits	4. Other vegetables & fruits	4. Breads & cereals
5. Leafy greens & yellow vegetables	5. Butter & fat	
6. Other vegetables and fruits	6. Lean meat, poultry & fish	
7. Eggs	7. Flour & cereals	
8. Lean meat, poultry, fish		
9. Flour and cereals		
10. Butter		
11. Other fat		
12. Sugars		

These ideas for a "balanced diet" were accepted by both the food industry and the medical profession. No one ever questioned them. People thought, "Well, food is food. It doesn't matter if we eat M&M's or an apple, we'll be healthy." Yet, it does matter. **As foods become less nutritious, every generation became weaker.**

As the *variety* of the food groups, including fruits and vegetables, *decreased,* our longevity also decreased. Rather than living years longer, the Basic Four plan almost guaranteed degenerative diseases.

Imagine if there were a "dietary standard" for Adam and Eve. It would probably be called, "The Genesis Diet," and would include fruits available in the Mediterranean area.

**The Genesis Diet
(Era of Adam and Eve)**

Fruit: Apples, pears, oranges, bananas, mangoes, grapes, grapefruit, kiwi, blueberries, raspberries, gooseberries, currants, apricots, peaches, plums, huckleberries, strawberries, figs, avocadoes, tomatoes and olives

---

Let's go a step further and write a dietary standard for Jesus and His disciples. It would probably be similar to our Old Basic Twelve, and called, "The Bread of Life Diet" and it would include foods available in the Mediterranean area.

**The Bread of Life Diet
(Era of Jesus and the Disciples)**

1. Milk such as yogurt, curds (cottage cheese)
2. Vegetables: cabbage, sweet potatoes, green leafy vegetables, carrots, cucumbers, and so on
3. Fruits: apples, pears, oranges, bananas, grapes, figs
4. Breads, pasta, brown rice, couscous, polenta, and other whole grains
5. Beans, legumes and nuts
6. Fats such as olive oil
7. Fish and poultry
8. Red meat (only during celebrations)
9. Sweets (only during celebrations)

Do you think that at the time of Jesus, the disciples were walking around saying to each other, "Hey, which diet are you going to follow this year? I'm thinking about the "Bread of Life Diet." No, they didn't have much choice! If you think about it, they probably didn't need any kind of "dietary standards" back then. Everything was organic and fresh! They didn't have the food processing methods that we have today. Everyone ate the same food, and people ate a whole foods diet, much like that of the Mediterranean area today. They had to go shopping every day. Milk didn't last a month in their refrigerator! (They didn't have refrigerators.) And there is much indication that they didn't eat three (or five or more!) times a day like we do. They probably only ate twice a day, in the morning and again later in the day.

They didn't gain weight because they walked everywhere in the universe! "We can't go see your Aunt Ester, until next month, Mary. We all have to get ready for the eight-day trip." Not everyone had camels back then.

Why do we need "dietary guides"? Because we have too much processed food, and too many choices. If we wanted, it would be possible to go an entire year without a fruit or vegetable! It's so bad that unfortunately, a typical teen's dietary standard might look like this:

A Teenager's "Basic Four" Food Groups
Year: 2004

Main Entre: Pizza

Beverage: Soda

Vegetables: French fries

Dessert: M&Ms

What have these standards done for us? "The Dietary Goals of the United States," showed us how these changes affected us:[11]

> The over-consumption of fat, generally, and saturated fat in particular, as well as cholesterol, sugar, salt and alcohol, have been related to six of the ten leading causes of death: Heart disease, cancer, cerebrovascular disease, diabetes, arteriosclerosis, and cirrhosis of the liver.

These changes created dietary imbalances which have damaged our nation's health. Only in the last twenty years have we understood the dangers of these "dietary standards" and their link to diabetes, heart disease, and cancer.

Why Moses and Grandma Lived Long

I'm often amazed at the genetic health of some of my elderly clients, yet if we look at how they grew up, we can understand why they are healthier than their children and grandchildren. They grew up with few, if any, chemicals and preservatives. The water was cleaner, the air was purer, and the soil was richer in minerals. Many of them worked hard on farms, and there were no fast-food restaurants. They were eating a variety of foods, and they ate more fruits and vegetables per person than any other generation. (Some of the foods that they consumed are now only sold in health food stores such as wheat germ and flaxseeds!)

If you are in your 40s or 50s, think about the foods you grew up on. I remember eating cold cereal (the first kind with the plastic toys inside the box), jello, TV dinners and Hamburger Helper. As bad as I ate, later generations are eating even worse, and each generation is getting sicker.

An Updated Food Group

It's no wonder that people are still confused. I recently had a client tell me that her idea of a "balanced diet" was a Twinkie in one hand and a soda in the other!

In the mid-1990s, the out-of-date "Basic Four" was replaced by the USDA Food Guide Pyramid (No, it doesn't have anything to do with Egypt, the Pyramids, or even the Mediterranean diet!) in an effort to bring balance to our former lopsided dietary guidelines. While this long overdue Food Guide Pyramid is better than the "Basic Four," unfortunately it still needs revision.

The Food Guide Pyramid increased the amount of carbohydrates to more than 6 to 11 servings a day, and decreased the amount of fat from 45 percent to 30 percent.

But some vital differences are not clear on the Food Guide Pyramid. For example, there is a big difference between a serving of whole-grain bread and processed white bread and between margarine and butter. Eating so many carbohydrates has made our health statistics even worse.

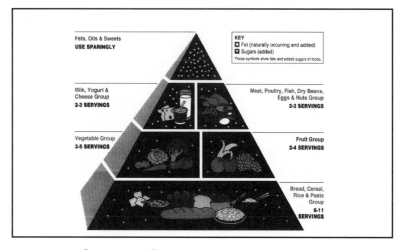

Anyone for Bread or Pasta?

Being a health nut, I began eating brown rice rather than white rice. My early bean-eating, rice-chewing days were good. However, after a period of time, I noticed that I didn't feel as good as I used to. Often, I ate toast and cereal for breakfast, whole-wheat sandwiches for lunch, and brown rice and vegetables for dinner. Unfortunately, I gained more weight and couldn't keep it off. In fact, I had worse sugar and carbohydrate cravings than before. I wasn't the only one who has struggled with carbohydrates. The average American eats 250-500 grams of carbohydrates a day (processed breads, cereals, pastas, pizzas, soda and fruit beverages each contain about 25 or more carbohydrate grams). We used to eat one-third or less of that amount. **Now, nearly half of our population is overweight, and about 13 percent of our children are overweight after following the high-carbohydrate, low-fat way of eating.** The Food Guide Pyramid isn't balanced. Yet it's still being taught to school children across the nation, while the incidence of diabetes in children continues to skyrocket.

A Better, Biblically-Based Guide

An organization named Oldways along with Harvard School of Public Health and other institutions, published a set of "healthy eating pyramids," unique dietary guides based on worldwide dietary traditions closely associated with good health. Separate pyramids have been made around Asian, Latin American, Mediterranean and Vegetarian diets.

These pyramids are welcome alternatives to the outdated Food Guide Pyramid and differ from it in many ways.

Unlike the Food Guide Pyramid, the Oldways pyramids represent actual traditional diets from cultures around the world—diets that have been scientifically proven to promote good health over the long term.

The Food Guide Pyramid recommends daily consumption of meat, despite research proving the health value of eating less red meat. Also, it combines beans, poultry, fish and nuts to a single "protein" food group, calling animal and plant protein as similar, which they are not.

The Oldways pyramid groups nuts, beans and legumes in one category and recommends their daily consumption along with vegetables and fruits. Fish and poultry are recommended only a few times a week; and meat is suggested only monthly or in small quantities.

Oldways recommends greater use of plant and vegetable oils (such as olive, peanut, and sesame oils) than of animal fats, while the Food Guide Pyramid lumps all fats and oils together, despite their great differences.

Unlike the Food Guide Pyramid, the Oldways pyramids recommend daily exercise as part of a healthy dietary routine.

The Mediterranean Food Pyramid is probably closer to how Jesus ate than any other. It describes Bible foods, includes the whole foods versions, and recommends daily physical activity. Here is the Mediterranean Food Pyramid: (used by permission of Oldways)[12]

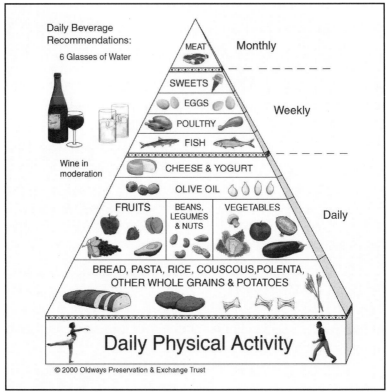

While I like the Mediterranean Food Pyramid, I would modify it this way:

1. Limit the number of whole grain servings to 3-4 a day.

2. Eat plenty of fruits, vegetables, beans and legumes, and only small amounts of olive oil, cheese and yogurt.

3. It's okay to eat eggs regularly if they are from free-range chickens.

4. Drink nonalcoholic wines and only eat natural sweet desserts.

We'll look again at the Mediterranean diet in chapter 10. So what about the foods we are eating then? Are they the same food that Jesus ate? Let's go on to look at how foods have become processed in America.

Chapter Four

New Giants on the Earth

Jesus never drank a Dr. Pepper. He never ate at McDonald's, and He never ate Krispy Kreme donuts! Thank God that "dietary standards" and junk foods weren't an issue back then. Jesus spent most of his ministry reaching the lost and teaching his followers. He didn't have to lobby the government of Israel about the foods people ate.

America is an affluent society, blessed with not only natural foods, but highly processed foods. In the last ten years, more than ten thousand "convenience processed foods" have been introduced in the United States. Although David killed Goliath, we still have giants on the earth. Paul Stitt, an author who spent years as a food scientist for two of the country's top corporations called the manufacturers of processed foods "Food Giants."

In his eye-opening book, *Beating the Food Giants,* Stitt talks about the casualties of processed food addiction which he calls "Can't Eat Just One Syndrome." What causes this syndrome and what's it doing to our bodies? Paul explains that Food Giants know if they add enough fat, sugar and salt, Americans will eat almost anything.[13]

> The real dirty tricks that food companies use to make you overeat are more subtle and don't jump out at you when you read the label—things like "natural flavoring"—which sounds very benign, but it can be almost anything, even suggesting that some ingredients have been known to contain monkey intestines. One thing for sure, it's there to make your taste buds go crazy so that if you eat just one bite, you're hooked and have to keep right on eating until the bag is empty.

Stitt writes that the most insidious, most misleading compounds ever added to foods are artificial sweeteners, because they're not added to make foods taste sweet; they're added to make you overeat. (If diet drinks worked, Americans would be the thinnest people on earth!) He explains that Nutrasweet didn't replace sugar; it increased the craving for sugar and the percentage of people overweight has increased. He further suggests you call the corporate research offices of Nutrasweet and ask them for some scientific proof that Nutrasweet has helped animals or humans lose weight. They don't have it because no controlled trial has ever proven that it works![14] Paul further wrote:

> Have you ever eaten just one Oreo cookie? Bet you can't either. They look so sweet and innocent! What you should realize is that the Nabisco Company spent millions developing that formula so that you can't eat just one. It contains 23 different appetite stimulants and 11 artificial colors. I saw the recipe and I was aghast. It's not easy to make a cookie that will hook every last American![15]

And you thought it was all because of your lack of willpower! Recently, I had some missionary clients who told me that when some of their African friends first tasted American junk food and soda, they spit it out, it was so foreign to their taste! Really, this should happen to us, too. You may remember a time when you stopped drinking soda or eating sugar, and then when you ate it again, it tasted bad!

Who Is Telling Us What To Eat?

Lisa Messinger, author of *Why Should I Eat Better?* tells us:[16]

> There is $400 billion floating around out there trying to get you to eat processed food, which is the largest industry in the United States. Food advertising is a $3.6 billion annual industry in this country, and almost a third of the ads include some type of "health" claim.

She later wrote that she attended a lecture where a lawyer gave tips to food technologists about how they could walk the fine line between puffery and out-and-out illegal deception in food product advertising![17]

Television has a major impact on everyone's lives. In her insightful book, *Train Up a Child in the Way They Should Eat,* Sharon Broer says that the television is telling our kids what to eat, day in and day out.[18] "Sandwiched between every seven-minute slice of The Power Rangers come a variety of thoroughly entertaining food commercials. With movie-quality sound, full-color animations and the highest tech production values, these ads tell our kids how good it'll feel to load up on junk."

She further writes:[19]

> The Boob-Tube doesn't tell you how bad it is for your child to be eating Fried Wonders, Sticky Goo-Goos and Creemie Cakes. Most of the loudly touted fare is little more than a colorful mixture of fat and sugar, usually with a "lucious cream-filled center." You might as well call your kids over to the kitchen counter, make them open wide and funnel a few quarts of sugar, lard, artificial flavors and dyes right into their bellies. Or give them a couple injections of melted Crisco.

How Did This Happen?

A *New York Times* article written by Marian Burros explains that the American Dietetic Association (ADA) takes the "wishy-washy stance" that there are not "good or bad foods," because they rely on food industry money which means that they never criticize the food industry. The ADA is funded by food companies.[20]

What you need to understand is that the ADA, which has more than 65,000 members, provides public education and sets nutritional guidelines for hospitals and schools. The ADA also receives substantial contributions from groups such as the National Livestock and Meat Board, Sugar Association, and from companies such as McDonald's, Coca-Cola, and other snack food companies.[21]

If there aren't any "bad" foods, why are we so sick and tired? We can't rely on "traditional, governmental" sources for our nutritional information when these sources are linked to the marketing of processed foods.

Are Additives Safe?

In the Bible days, food was often preserved naturally somewhat like our grandparents preserved food with salt and vinegar. That way, they could store food from one season to another. Today, the main reason food processors preserve food is to gain a longer shelf life. It's possible that some processed foods have longer shelf lives than Americans!

Want to know what they are putting in our food? The term "artificial colorings" actually refers to acidic dyes. In his book, *Pure & Simple Natural Weight Control,*[22] Dr. Norman Walker explains that Benzene, for example, is an ingredient used in coloring beverages. It's also used as a motor fuel and in the manufacturing of dyes. It's harmful because it adversely affects the nervous system and cerebrospinal fluid.

Dr. Walker also writes that sodium phosphate is a dye and coloring agent for beverages which interferes with the body's endocrine functioning. And tartrazine is a poisonous chemical also used as a coloring agent in beverages and foods. Flavorings are equally harmful, too. To learn more about the various chemicals in our food and what they can do to you, I recommend reading his book.[23]

George Malkmus explains in his book, *Why Christians Get Sick,* that along with chemical preservatives, artificial colorings and flavorings, stabilizers, emulsifiers are also used. On top of that, over one billion pounds of insecticides are sprayed or dusted on our foods. Unfortunately, many of these insecticides are hard to remove by washing or peeling since they become part of the plant. Pesticides can damage your immune system.[24]

An Attempt to Help

In response to public fears about food safety, Congress did try to regulate the food industry by passing the Delaney Clause, first introduced in 1958. It was originally written to forbid the sale of food containing a substance shown to produce cancer in laboratory animals or humans. What happened then?

Rather than taking dangerous chemicals off the market, things got worse. Author and Certified Nutritionist Carol Simontacchi wrote in her book called *Crazy Makers: How the Food Industry Is Destroying Our Brains and Harming Our Children*: "As a result of Delaney, the U.S. Food and Drug Administration and industry researchers aimed their efforts and money at proving that food additives are benign in terms of producing cancer."[25]

Three thousand chemicals are added to our foods daily. These chemicals are "man-made" in a laboratory and are foreign to our bodies. Instead of adding health and vitality, they are causing a greater burden on the immune system and filter systems. Additionally, no one has ever studied the cumulative effect of all of these food additives and preservatives on our bodies. We thought the FDA was looking out for us, but they don't have the time or resources to test the thousands of additives on the market.

Where Should We Turn?

Carol says that virtually everything written about nutrition in the mainstream press is wrong and potentially harmful. In her introduction she writes:[26]

> During the past century, food-processing companies and their creative marketers have changed the definition and composition of our food. Marketing efforts have been so successful that we no longer think it strange or even unhealthy to drink a liter of Coca-Cola per day instead of water.

The largest manufacturing industry in America is processed foods, and industry influences research studies. According to researcher Sally Fallon, universities have powerful ties to the food processing industry. She cites Dr. Frederick Stare, from the nutrition department at Harvard University as a good example. Early on, he wrote several articles implicating vegetable oils—not animal fats—as one of the major causes of heart disease. After he became department head, the university received several grants from the food processing industries. After that, his articles said that there was nothing wrong with white bread, sugar and processed foods. He even suggested Coca-Cola as a snack food![27]

What Have They Done To Our Food?

1. Food manufacturers add more than 3,000 chemicals to our foods, most of which have never been tested.

2. The meat industry uses drugs, hormones and antibiotics to raise animals faster.

3. The food processing industry strips natural foods of vitamins, fiber and minerals to process food.

4. Farmers fail to properly fertilize the soil with organic matter and trace minerals as was done in Biblical times.

Paul Stitt explains that to make diet foods, they put less food into a serving. For example, diet cheese has more air and water pumped into it than regular cheese, so each serving has less cheese. So they can now announce their foods have half the calories. To add insult to injury, the Food Giants charge substantially more for these flimsy "diet foods" than they charge for their regular products![28]

What Do Processed Foods Do?

Processed foods cause addictions! I've met: "Sugarholics," "Chocoholics," "Carbaholics," "Pastaholics," "Pizzaholics," "French fryaholics," "Bagelaholics," but so far, no "Saladaholics" or "Appleaholics!" Why? We aren't "addicted" to good food, because it "feeds" us fiber and many nutrients. You could probably eat several slices of white bread at one sitting, but you wouldn't be able to eat as many slices of real, unprocessed whole-grain bread because of the fiber. Fiber fills us up. We overeat "dead, processed" foods because they don't "feed" us nutrients, they only satisfy our taste buds, but don't fill us up.

Processed foods also stifle our children's physical and mental potential. I recently received an email from one of my clients named Mary who is a school teacher. She wrote:

> After the food inventory was taken today of each child's eating for twenty-four hours, it's not surprising why they can't sit in their seats without twitching and moving around and why they don't test well. One little girl drinks Dr. Pepper with every meal along with a white biscuit for breakfast, macaroni and cheese for lunch, and a grilled cheese sandwich for dinner, along with a snack of chocolate cookies. It's no wonder why she has "brain fog" and can't take a test!

Carol Simontacchi explains that we need whole foods, even when we are in the womb. She writes that when a woman is pregnant, it's vital that she get enough nutrition:[29]

> Lacking optimum nutrition during this period may mean that the child will never reach his or her genetic potential, that the brain or certain portions of the brain may not develop adequately. Genetics is an important factor in mental competency, but in the face of undernutrition or malnutrition, genetics is handcuffed.

Carol further shows us what happens to women when they eat processed foods while they are pregnant: "We eat nutrient dead food, food devoid of materials needed to develop into brains of our growing babies, and then wonder why our babies cry so much or seem so restless."[30]

Processed foods adversely affect behavior. Barbara Stitt, a Ph.D. in nutrition who studied nutrition and behavior in the prison system for years makes a solid case for reversing and preventing criminal violence with proper nutrition, in her book, *Food and Behavior*:[31]

> What is important for parents to know is that by doing something very basic and simple—by making sure that your kids are well nourished—you can make progress toward solving the problems of criminality, delinquency, violence and mental illness, and even help reduce the tremendous toll that crime and the attempted rehabilitation of convicts takes on the resources of society.

For years, we could rely on our natural wisdom to protect us from eating foods that would harm us. What happened? According to Paul Stitt:[32]

> The Food Giants and the medical establishment have had a big hand in it. The food industry started things off by destroying our knowledge of what is good to eat... The industry has spent billions of dollars encouraging us to link positive mental images with products that can only make us sick. It is little wonder that most of us have no idea of what truly good food is.

> The medical establishment, and especially the major over-the-counter drug manufacturers, strike a second blow by convincing us that every pain or ache or discomfort we feel is to be feared and suppressed.

For example, he asks:

> Does the commercial tell you to eat sensibly and inform you that indigestion is a sign that you are doing damage to your digestive tract? No—just take Pepto-Bismol and carry on. And the drug industry doesn't stop there. They've turned us into a nation of pill poppers.

What must God think about how we have adulterated His food! We are eating foods that Jesus and His disciples never ate and never imagined. I like what Dr. Patrick Quillin says in his book, *Healing Secrets From the Bible*:[33]

> Every time we think that we can improve on nature, we find our confidence misplaced. Every time we fiddle with a wholesome food, we erode its nutrient value. In whole foods lies a universe of nutrients that we will never fully understand but are Divinely placed there for our benefit.

> Food is a rich tapestry of thousands of substances. Foods contain life giving agents that we are only beginning to understand.

> God is the ultimate engineer in designing and building the human body and providing us with all our needs. When we tamper with the food supply, we usually wreak havoc on the food's nutritional content.

Let's now look at what the Food Giants do to process foods, starting with sugar.

Chapter Five

How Much Is a "Little" Honey?

Have you ever wondered what Jesus and the disciples snacked on? Do you suppose they had Hershey bar trees or M&M shrubs? How about licorice on the vine?

I imagine they snacked on dried figs and fruits. Okay, maybe someone in their town knew how to make that delicious dessert, Baklava! After all, it was made with honey. But surely they only had it occasionally. During the thousands of years of human evolution, our ancestors survived fine without any other sugar other than those occurring in wild fruits and berries. (And my clients have trouble going a day without sugar!)

You and I may have grown up eating refined white sugar, but did you know that chemically refined white sugar is fairly recent? According to Mary June Parks in *Will Bible Foods Prevent Cancer?*, for centuries, sugar was sold by the teaspoonful only through drug stores. Originally crude, unrefined beet sugar was a luxury.[34]

The word "sugar" is not in the Bible, and has actually only been used in the last hundred years. A comparable Bible food was honey, which has more than 50 scripture references. But Proverbs 25:27 warns us: *It is not good to eat much honey.*

In 1975, *Sugar Blues* by William Dufty, (a book still in print) made us aware of the dangers of refined sugar, calling it a poison.[35] In the 1800s, the average American ate about 10 pounds of sugar per year. Today, individual consumption of sugar has skyrocketed, especially with the increase in low-fat or fat-free products which contain large amounts of "hidden" sugar. Today the average American consumes about 200 pounds of sugar per person, per year!

It's no wonder that diabetes is one of the fastest-growing diseases with more than 2,000 people being diagnosed daily. According to the American Diabetes Association, in the U.S., approximately 16 million people have diabetes. The incidence of diabetes has increased six-fold since 1930. The risk for heart disease and stroke increases tremendously when a person has diabetes.

But I Don't Eat Sugar!

You may not buy it intentionally, but sugar is everywhere! Of course you already knew sugar is in cookies, ice cream, candy, and pop. But did you know it's the number-one food additive hidden in salad dressings, mayonnaise, peanut butter, pickles, canned fruits and vegetables, breads, crackers, ketchups, spaghetti sauce, soups, cereals, luncheon meats, pizza, and juices?

You may not recognize that a product has sugar in it because of its many different names. Raw, natural, yellow D, cane sugar, brown sugar, caramel, corn fructose, corn sweetener, corn syrup, dextrose, high fructose corn syrup, and white sugar are all sucrose.

They can all become addictive and are empty calories. Here is an explanation of three common types of sugars:

Dextrose is a refined crystalline sugar which is 99.9% sucrose.

Refined corn syrup is a liquified version of dextrose used to sweeten hundreds of commercial food products.

Refined high fructose corn syrup is another type of refined syrup which is 20% sweeter than sucrose and cheaper. It's still 99.9 % sucrose.

Product ingredients are listed on the label in descending order by weight, from the greatest to the least. So if one of these sugars is listed as one of the first three ingredients, or if there are several sugars listed, the product is high in sugar.

The U.S. Department of Agriculture recommends only 10 teaspoons of refined sugar every day, but many nutritionists consider two teaspoons per day too much. Consider that the average American eats about 20 or more teaspoons per day. That total is the amount of sugar only. It doesn't take into consideration the amount of processed carbohydrates like white bread and pasta which turn to sugar in the body.

How Can We Eat That Much Sugar?

For example, my friend and teacher, Dr. Michael Dobbins shows how we can easily get 3-5 cups of sugar in the daily average American diet:

Breakfast: Cereal, white toast, orange juice and banana: 1 cup sugar.

Lunch: Yogurt with fruit, baked potato, white bread and chicken: 3/4 cup sugar.

3:00 snack: candy bar and soda: 1 1/2 cup sugar.

Dinner: Pasta, white bread, soda: 1 3/4 cup sugar.

Three cups of sugar translates to about 24 teaspoons of sugar. But did you realize that one can of soda alone can contain between 10 to 14 teaspoons of sugar?

Author and Certified Nutritionist Carol Simontacchi says that teens consume the most sugar:[36]

> Consider the common figures we all hear about—how the average American eats over two hundred pounds of sugar and artificial sweeteners per year (over twenty teaspooons per day). The average teenager guzzles twice as much soft drink as milk, but young adults from their twenties to their thirties drink nearly three times more than that. The typical teenage male who drinks soda, drinks over forty-two ounces every day, and the habits of girls are only slightly better.

But what about school lunches? Carol reports:

> Parents today can't count on school districts to help teach their children good nutritional habits. People managing the school... earn millions of dollars each year by inviting fast-food chains and soft drink dispensers into schools.
>
> Schools end up teaching that it's okay to drink pop instead of water, to eat candy bars instead of fresh fruit, to load up the

body on artificial this and that....as long as money can be made. Meanwhile, students' test scores are dropping, and the administrations cry out for more funding.

Soft drinks also pull vital minerals from the bones and cause an imbalance of phosphorus and calcium in the body which eventually can be responsible for the stiffening of joints and limbs in arthritic conditions. Our teenagers are drinking more soft drinks than ever. That's why our young people are starting to develop health and weight problems much earlier in life. I'm shocked at the number of young people who have come into my office with arthritis, diabetes, and weight problems.

Simple sugars like those found in fruit are good. In its natural form, sugar cane is a rich source of vitamins and minerals. But simple sugars which have been processed from sugar cane, beets or fruits and even further refined are dangerous. Let's look at several reasons why.

Sugar Is Bad (And That's Not Good!)

Years ago, I heard Dr. Patrick Quillin, nutritionist and former director of the Cancer Treatment Center in Tulsa, say that after drinking a can of soda, our immune system is depressed for the next 6-8 hours!

Refined sugar excess upsets the mineral balance in your body. Processed white sugar depletes precious vitamins, minerals, fibers and enzymes, so the body depletes its own store of these minerals and coenzymes in order to metabolize the sugar. Minerals that we need to handle sugar are chromium, magnesium and manganese. To make matters worse, many of these minerals, and especially chromium, are deficient in much of America's not-so-rich soil. The result of a chromium deficiency? Continual cravings for—you guessed it—more sugar!

I recommend people take nutritional supplements such as chromium and zinc which help them not crave sugar while they are changing their diet.

Paul Bragg, in *Healthful Eating Without Confusion,* wrote about the relationship between sugar and heart disease:[37]

> To clinch the argument that refined white sugar rather than fats is to blame for many of modern man's degenerative diseases, anthropologist Dr. Robert McCracken cited certain primitive tribes who consume many more saturated fats than Western man, but who never touch refined white sugar or its products. These people have very low blood cholesterol levels, and very few of the diseases to which we in the West fall victim. He calls refined white sugar "the worst thing man can eat."

Sugar Is Not a Health Food

And ladies, eating a diet high in refined white sugar can also make you look and feel older, age faster, and cause dandruff, wrinkles, and skin problems!

Here is a list of 78 ways that sugar can ruin your health from Nancy Appleton author of the book, *Lick the Sugar Habit.* Her web page, www.nancyappleton.com, lists each of the references which are based on scientific literature. I have acquired permission to publish her list because I think it's so important to understand that sugar is at the root of our fatigue, as well as most degenerative diseases.[38]

Sugar can:

1. Suppress the immune system.
2. Upset the body's mineral balance.
3. Cause hyperactivity, anxiety, concentration difficulties, and crankiness in children.
4. Cause drowsiness and decreased activity in children.
5. Adversely affect children's school grades.
6. Produce a significant rise in triglycerides.
7. Contribute to a weakened defense against bacterial infection.
8. Cause kidney damage.
9. Reduce helpful high density cholesterol (HDLs).
10. Promote an elevation of harmful cholesterol (LDLs).
11. Lead to chromium deficiency.
12. Cause copper deficiency.
13. Interfere with absorption of calcium and magnesium.
14. Lead to cancer of the breast, ovaries, prostate, and rectum.

15. Cause colon cancer, with an increased risk in women.
16. Be a risk factor in gall bladder cancer.
17. Increase fasting levels of blood glucose.
18. Weaken eyesight.
19. Raise the level of a neurotransmitter called serotonin, which can narrow blood vessels.
20. Cause hypoglycemia.
21. Produce an acidic stomach.
22. Raise adrenaline levels in children.
23. Increase the risk of coronary heart disease.
24. Speed the aging process, causing wrinkles and grey hair.
25. Lead to alcoholism.
26. Promote tooth decay.
27. Contribute to weight gain and obesity.
28. Increase the risk of Crohn's disease and ulcerative colitis.
29. Cause a raw, inflamed intestinal tract in persons with gastric or duodenal ulcers.
30. Cause arthritis
31. Cause asthma.
32. Cause candidiasis (yeast infection).
33. Lead to the formation of gallstones.
34. Lead to the formation of kidney stones.
35. Cause ischemic heart disease.
36. Cause appendicitis.
37. Exacerbate the symptoms of multiple sclerosis.
38. Indirectly cause hemorrhoids.
39. Cause varicose veins.
40. Elevate glucose and insulin responses in oral contraception users.
41. Lead to periodontal disease.
42. Contribute to osteoporosis.
43. Contribute to saliva acidity.
44. Cause a decrease in insulin sensitivity.
45. Lead to decreased glucose tolerance.
46. Decrease growth hormone.
47. Increase total cholesterol.
48. Increase systolic blood pressure.
49. Change the structure of protein causing interference with protein absorption.

50. Cause food allergies.
51. Contribute to diabetes.
52. Cause toxemia during pregnancy.
53. Contribute to eczema in children.
54. Cause cardiovascular disease.
55. Impair the structure of DNA.
56. Cause cataracts.
57. Cause emphysema.
58. Cause atherosclerosis.
59. Cause free radical formation in the bloodstream.
60. Lower the enzyme's ability to function.
61. Cause loss of tissue elasticity and function.
62. Cause liver cells to divide, increasing the size of the liver.
63. Increase the amount of fat in the liver.
64. Increase kidney size and produce pathological changes in the kidney.
65. Overstress the pancreas, causing damage.
66. Increase the body's fluid retention.
67. Cause constipation.
68. Cause myopia (nearsightedness).
69. Compromise the lining of the capillaries.
70. Cause hypertension.
71. Cause headaches, including migraines.
72. Cause an increase in delta, alpha and theta brain waves, which can alter the mind's ability to think clearly.
73. Cause depression.
74. Increase insulin responses in those consuming high-sugar diets compared to low-sugar diets.
75. Increase bacterial fermentation in the colon.
76. Cause hormonal imbalance.
77. Increase blood platelet adhesiveness which increases risk of blood clots.
78. Increase the risk of Alzheimer's Disease.

While the sugar industry denies that sugar is hazardous to human health, I'm looking forward to the day when foods will be labeled according to what they do to us. Here's one for sugar: "This is a diabetes-inducing, fat-storing, and disease-producing substance. Eating this food may make you crave sweets, increase your risk of heart disease, and make you fat!"

Why Is There Violence In Our Schools?

Burgess Parks, Mary June Park's husband, spent 32 years as a public school administrator. When he retired in 1970, there were only isolated cases of violence in schools. Today violence in schools is rampant. But no one is asking about their students' diets. In *Will Bible Foods Prevent Cancer?*, she reports that when they checked into the diets of juvenile delinquents, it was always "sugar-laden junk food." High amounts of sugar and soda burn up the B complex vitamins. Symptoms of a serious B vitamin deficiency are: anxiety, depression, mental confusion, insanity, irritability, and rage.[39]

Barbara Stitt's research concludes that sugar consumption leads to hypoglycemia and thus leads to aberrant and often violent behavior. She explains that sugar consumption causes nutrient depletion. Foods highest in sugar are lowest in vitamins. Sugar contains no micronutrients, yet in order to be turned into energy, it uses up a wide range of nutrients. So foods high in sugar provide little or no nutrition and actually rob nutrients from the body. Sugar consumption causes damage to brain function by causing hypoglycemia and contributing to nutrient depletion.[40]

Barbara also says, "I am convinced that if we could eradicate hypoglycemia, many other mental illnesses and behavioral disorders would take care of themselves."[41]

How Sugar Is Refined

Sugar cane stalks are cut, crushed, washed, boiled, steamed, and then crystallized. Finally, they are filtered, cleaned and decolorized. Lime, acids and bleaching agents are added until it becomes the white, "pure" substance we recognize as sugar. This product is so different from its original form that our bodies don't even recognize refined sugar as a food! No wonder it can give us a tummy ache!

All Sugars Are Not Created Equal!

Aspartame is found in about 5,000 products and it accounts for more than 80% of FDA food related complaints. Aspartame is 200 times sweeter than sugar and has been used to take the place of saccharin in foods and drinks. Its major brand names are NutraSweet and Equal. It has been linked to PKU seizures, high blood pressure, headaches, insomnia, and mood swings. Several studies have shown immediate serious reactions to aspartame: Severe headaches, extreme dizziness, throat swelling, and other allergic effects, including retina deterioration. And the worse thing is that these sweeteners don't satisfy our sweet tooth. (Remember, having a sweet tooth is a sign of a chromium or zinc deficiency, or other blood-sugar imbalance.)

Saccharin is one of the common forms of sugar substitutes known as Sweet-N-Low, Sprinkle Sweet, Sugar Twin, and Sweet 10. It comes from petroleum and is 300 times sweeter than sugar. Although the FDA proposed a ban on saccharin after studies suggested a link between it and tumors in rats, it was saved by public demand for it and was left on the market. Its safety is under review.

Notice the warning on the back of the saccharin packet: "Use of this product may be hazardous to your health. This product contains saccharin which has been determined to cause cancer in laboratory animals." Many other countries have banned artificial sweeteners because of their link to cancer risk.

A popular artificial sweetener used in low-carb foods is called Splenda. For a list of reasons why you should hesitate to use it, see www.mercola.com.

Natural, Healthy Sweet Alternatives

When natural foods like honey and maple syrup are heated over 130° F. the enzymes are killed and processing makes them more like processed white sugar. So the thing to look at is not only the type of sugar, but how it's processed. Below is a list of these natural, healthy alternatives and how you can use them.

Raw, unfiltered honey is twice as sweet as sugar and should be avoided by diabetics, hypoglycemics, and people with Candida. It's tempting to replace sugar with honey, but honey is still high in calories. Raw honey does however, contain many vitamins and enzymes and has some antibiotic properties. For centuries, honey was used as a medicine to help harmonize the liver, neutralize toxins, and relieve pain. Honey is used to treat sore throats, ulcers, high blood pressure, and constipation.

Try honey wherever you would normally use sugar. For example, use it on cereal, in baked recipes, and in hot drinks.

Sucanat is one of the best sweeteners to substitute for refined white sugar. Similar to brown sugar, but healthier, Sucanat is a dried granulated cane juice which contains all the vitamins, minerals, and trace elements from sugar cane. It's made by squeezing the juice from sugar cane and then evaporating the water. It's used one-to-one in place of sugar and works great in baked goods like breads and muffins.

The herb stevia is a wonderful natural sweetener and is used safely by diabetics. Stevia is a small plant that grows in Latin America. It's been used for centuries by the Indians of Brazil and Paraguay to sweeten tea. The Japanese consume more stevia than any other country in the world, and stevia now has wide commercial value in Japan to sweeten toothpaste, soft drinks, chewing gum, frozen desserts, and other foods. It's 200-300 times sweeter than sugar, yet it doesn't upset the blood sugar level. That's why it is successfully used by diabetics. It helps control sugar cravings, and unlike sucrose and fructose, will not feed Candida yeast.

Xylitol has recently received a lot of press. It's a natural extract from corn cobs that looks and tastes like sugar. It's also slower to cause an insulin response and may help prevent cavities. The only downside is that it's quite expensive.

Let's now look at how the Food Giants process our grains.

Chapter Six

Why Jesus Didn't Eat White Bread

Imagine how life would have been if the Food Giants had been around in Bible days. Instead of whole-grain breads, they would have eaten white bread. And think about how it might have affected the disciples. Paul, for example, when he boasted of the hardships he endured in 1 Cor. 11:24-27, might have added: "And for eight days, I was constipated!"

The words "bread" and "food" were practically interchangeable in the Bible. Even a quick read of the Bible tells us that there are more references to bread than any other food. Whole grains and bread were staples for Jesus and the disciples. Jesus was called the "Bread of Life," and the Lord's prayer began with, *Give us this day our daily bread* (Matt. 6).

Scriptural history (Genesis 41-43) shows when there was a great famine in the land, the key food was grain that was stored for seven years. Most other foods perish quickly. Whole grains however will last indefinitely. Archaeologists have found whole grain from ancient Egyptian tombs that could still be sprouted.

Today, though, people are cutting back and even entirely eliminating bread. Yet I can't imagine Jesus going on a low-carb diet! What has happened to our precious "daily bread?" Let's look at how processing has changed Bible grains.

Types of Bible Grains

- Barley
- Brown rice
- Buckwheat
- Wheat
- Millet
- Rye
- Oat Bran
- Oatmeal

In Bible days, grains like barley and wheat were a staple; barley was eaten by the common man, yet it is extremely nutritious. Wheat was the choice for the nobility.

High-fiber complex carbohydrates like whole grains have always been valuable in traditional, long-lived cultures. These whole grain foods are high in vitamins, minerals, and fiber. No wonder these traditional cultures can remain so healthy! Remember, natural complex carbohydrates are low in fat, high in fiber, and nutrient dense—which means they contain a high ratio of nutrients per calorie.

You are probably familiar with brown rice, oat bran, and oatmeal. Millet is a small round grain, the kind that is often used in bird seed! There's also buckwheat (nice in pancakes), barley (which makes nice breads and soups), and rye. Whole wheat is hard to eat as a whole grain, but is often used as a flour in whole-wheat bread, or whole-wheat cereals.

What's On Their Plate?

Cereal grains and vegetable foods have been one of man's chief dietary staples through the ages. Rice was used by the Indians and Orientals; corn was used by the Mexicans and North and South Americans, and wheat was used by the Russians, Argentineans and North and South Americans.

The high-fiber Hunza diet of Pakistan, consists of whole grains, vegetables, and fruit. Millet, one of their staple grains, is high in protein. They eat a majority of their food raw because they can't easily cook food. Many researchers believe that their diet of ordinary whole foods is the cause for their incredible health and longevity.

The Tarahumara Indians of Mexico eat a diet of complex carbohydrates consisting of corn, squash, beans, peas and fruit, and a small amount of animal protein about once a month, or 12 times a year. They have no obesity, heart disease, hypertension and/or diabetes.

According to health researcher and author, Paul Bragg:[42]

54

Records of the Spanish conquistadores, which have been preserved in the archives of Spain and which I have studied with great care, show that this native corn (maize) was also important in the diet of the highly advanced civilizations of the Aztecs and Mayans centuries ago. The Spaniards reported that these races were healthy, powerful people, free of disease. They found no bald headed men, and no retarded or congenitally crippled children. There were no insane persons, no premature aging, no decayed teeth. Their bodies, both young and matured, were things of beauty.

Bragg further wrote:[43]

The rice eating people of Asia have survived hardily for thousands of years with natural brown rice as their basic food. But when they started using civilized white rice, which has lost its coat that contains the B complex and other important vitamins, minerals and nutrients, their health degenerated. In Hawaii, there are many Orientals. The preponderance of these people use devitalized white rice as the basic item in their diet. As a result, much of their money and time is spent in hospitals, clinics, doctors and dentists, because of sick bodies and decaying teeth.

Where's the Milk, Fat and Sugar?

Americans think of carbohydrates as either pasta and bread or if they are more health minded, they think of whole-grain breads and pastas. Most traditional cultures ate a cereal grain which was eaten as a main dish or porridge rather than bread. The bread that they did eat was not like our breads. They baked corn tortillas, whole-grain wheat chapatis or barley cakes. These are yeast-free flat breads, made with little salt and oil. No processed muffins or white breads were on their menu. They really had to chew, chew, chew! No wonder they didn't gain weight; these breads were so hearty that I imagine one piece was enough. Even our homemade whole-wheat breads were not as nutrient rich as theirs.

A common denominator in the healthy diets of traditional cultures and the diets of people in Bible days is fiber. Fiber is the indigestible remnant in fruits, vegetables, nuts, seeds, beans, peas and whole grains that is not broken down. Fiber is found mainly in plant based foods; animal foods like meat, fish, poultry and dairy do not have fiber.

The Whole Grain and Nothing But the Grain

There are three main parts of any whole grain: 1) The bran, which is the outer layer; 2) The germ or inside of the base of the grain; and 3) The endosperm or the starch in the center.

A whole grain refers to the entire grain—the bran, the germ, and the endosperm. Processing whole grains separates the bran and germ which are both necessary to digest the starch. God never made a starch without all the parts, and grains were health foods. Here's why:

The fiber protects us against colon cancer, and the germ protects us against heart disease.

Prevent Cancer With Fiber

It is estimated that one out of three people will get cancer of the colon. That's not hard to imagine, when we consider that the average American diet still consists of hamburgers, white bread, mashed potatoes with gravy, pancakes made with white flour, smothered with syrup, peanut butter and jelly on white bread, French fries, and few, if any, vegetables!

Grandma isn't the only one touting fiber. The 1988 Surgeon General's report stated that we needed to reduce the intake of foods high in fat and increase foods high in complex carbohydrates and fiber. There is a definite parallel between the increase of colon and gastrointestinal disorders and the decrease in dietary fiber. That's why the National Cancer Institute, American Cancer Society and American Heart Association recommend that we increase our fiber intake from our typical 7-10 grams to 35-40 grams.

Dr. Don Colbert, wrote in his book, *Walking in Divine Health,* that we don't have to get cancer or heart disease:[44]

Colon cancer, the second leading cause of cancer death, is at epidemic proportions in our country because of two reasons: The percentage of pesticides and toxins we are taking into our bodies; the low fiber content of the foods we eat. The solution lies in eating fruits and vegetables that contain enough fiber to help bind toxins and eliminate them from the colon.

Traditional cultures eat almost four times more fiber than we do—forty, sixty and even one hundred grams per day. The common denominator for all of those healthy cultures we discussed earlier was the amount of fiber they ate. No wonder they have lower rates of disease.

How Enriched Is Flour?

Whole-wheat flours and breads can't keep as long, but you can simply store them in the freezer or refrigerator. The vitamin E in whole-wheat flour acts as an antioxidant to prevent rancidity too.

You may wonder about the history of enriched flour. In the 1940s, public health officials tried for years to get people to switch back to whole-wheat flour because of a severe outbreak of pellagra and beri-beri, two diseases which could be prevented by B vitamins found in wheat bran. But people were resistant to change, so the government added an "enrichment" compound of synthetic B vitamins to their refined wheat, corn, and rice.

Yet these flours were not very enriched.

Did you know that up to 70 percent of the essential nutrients are lost in the production of white flour? After white flour is rolled, it's then bleached by chlorine dioxide where any vitamin E is completely destroyed. In the refinement process, more than 21 nutrients are taken out, and only a handful are put back in.

Even as far back as 1942, a nutrition-minded dentist named Dr. Royal Lee was calling for legislative action to protect the public health against these vitamin and nutrient deficiencies when he said:[45]

No food is safe unless it is fresh enough to retain its perishable vitamins, incurred no processing that would remove or impair its vitamin and mineral content; free of any kind of synthetic adulteration, and unless it has a background of experience behind it establishing its value to the human family.

Prevent Heart Disease With Whole Grains

There is so much evidence of the correlation between heart disease and white flour that Dr. Lee said, **"We might as well remove the term heart disease and supplant it with 'white-flour disease.'"**[46]

Dr. Lee said that a better way to make flour is to grind it with stone buhrs to as fine a degree as possible; then sift out the major part of the fibrous remainder. This retains the complete germ portion of the wheat. Of course, he added that since this flour requires refrigeration, manufacturers would have to use vacuum-packed tins.[47]

According to Paul Stitt:[48]

Wheat flour is especially ravaged by processing. In the refining process, more than half of each of the most essential nutrients is sold for making pet food. The milling process destroys 40% of the chromium present in the whole grain, as well as 86% of the manganese, 89% of the cobalt, 68% of the copper, 78% of the zinc, and 48% of the molybdenum. By the time it is completely refined, it has lost most of its phosphorus, iron, and thiamine, and a good deal of its niacin and riboflavin. Its crude fiber content has been cut down considerably as well. Yet all of these nutrients are needed for a healthy body.

Stitt says that the history of the food industry is replete with examples of this constant and insidious process. It was the introduction of pre-sweetened cereals, for example, which saved a flagging cereal market in 1948, and the Food Giants learned that the more sugar they added to their products, the better they sold. Bread manufacturers also learned that white bread sold better than whole grain bread.[49] But at what cost?

The high heat and pressure used in the processing of puffed grains also makes the grains toxic. In his book, Paul Stitt reported an experiment where rats were fed whole wheat or puffed wheat. The rats who ate the whole wheat lived more than a year, while the rats that ate the puffed wheat died within two weeks.[50]

The more you eat processed white flour foods, the more you crave them. We eat between 250-500 grams of carbohydrates a day, and most of them are made from processed white flour, without the protective parts. The result: Obesity has increased 30%, cravings are rampant, and heart disease and diabetes have skyrocketed.

Eat unprocessed, unrefined carbohydrates packed with fiber. But limit them to a reasonable amount. Most of my clients do well eating 2 or 3 servings a day of whole-grain foods rather than the recommended 6-12 in the Food Guide Pyramid.

Perhaps one of the easiest ways to increase your fiber intake is to eat legumes, nuts, seeds, vegetables, fruits and whole grains—which all contain good plant based fiber.

Label Reading 101

Relying on commercially-prepared fiber cereals isn't the answer, though. It's no surprise that most kid's breakfast cereals have fructose, corn syrup, and fat; it's like eating candy bars for breakfast! These cereals were designed to satisfy their taste buds but not their bodies. Many of these foods actually have little fiber, so a good rule of thumb is to purchase cereals with at least 4-6 grams of fiber per serving.

Teach your children how to eat properly at a young age. When children grow up having eaten "real" foods, sugared, processed foods cereals and snacks taste artificial to them.

When shopping for breads and cereals, read labels! Just because the label says "wheat bread" and comes in a brown label doesn't mean that it's really made from whole grains. Many of these bread labels, for example, which say "multi grain" or "cracked wheat," usually contain far more white flour than anything else. By law, bread that is labeled whole wheat must be made from 100% whole-wheat flour. Wheat bread may be made from varying proportions of white and wheat flour. The type of flour used is listed first on the label.

Sometimes a dark color is provided by using caramel coloring, which is also listed on the label. A rip off again folks! Remember, a healthy, whole-grain bread spoils in a few days. Unless you are buying breads that are in the freezer section, they are probably not whole-grain breads.

Many commercial products, both crackers, breads and cereals are still high in fat, sugar and preservatives. It's far better to eat a variety of fruits, vegetables, whole grains, and legumes and even take a fiber supplement than to eat these processed foods.

Start Slowly

Changing suddenly from a low-fiber to a high-fiber diet may cause serious problems in the intestines. A sudden shift to a high-fiber diet may cause impactions of the bowel wall. Here is a good way to start:

1. Substitute whole grain brown rice for white rice.

2. Eat 1-2 fruits and 4-5 vegetables daily.

3. Eat a high-fiber cereal with at least four to six grams of dietary fiber per ounce of cereal. Oat bran cereal is better than oatmeal.

4. Add 3 or 4 servings of beans or legumes to your weekly menus.

5. Add other whole grain products like oats, millet or barley.

6. Substitute whole-grain flours like wheat, brown rice flour or oat flour for white flour. (My friend, Linda, grinds up her own oats and uses oat flour to make gravy, desserts, and pie crusts.)

7. Take a digestive aid or product like beano when eating high roughage foods.

Okay, let's now look at what Food Giants do to our fats and proteins.

Chapter Seven

We're Supposed to Eat Fat!

God made us with a desire to eat and enjoy fat! I've tried no-fat diets, and you probably have, too. After a few days, you begin to look for oil for your salad and butter for your bread! Going no-fat was no fun!

Jesus and His crew didn't have fat gram counters. In fact, they didn't need to count fats, carbohydrates or calories. Because of God's Word, they naturally ate the right fats.

In the Bible, God gave strict orders about the animal fat that they could eat. God instructed the Israelites to burn the fat that surrounded the organs in animal meat as an offering to the Lord (it was not for the people to eat). *...Ye shall eat neither fat nor blood* (Leviticus 3:17). This fat—lard, bacon fat and shortening—is not only hard to digest, but also is the animal fat known to cause health problems.

But good fats are essential for health. There are essential amino acids. This means there are certain amino acids that our body doesn't make, that we must obtain from outside sources—our diet. The same is true of fats. Some fats are essential because they are not made by our body, but they are required through food or supplementation. And in recent years, research has shown the importance of these fats in our diets. We desperately need some good fat.

When your body is fat-starved, you become hungry and overeat, often binging on carbohydrates and sweets. Many people think they have a "sweet tooth," when in fact, they may have a "fat tooth." What they really want when they think they want sweets is fat. For example, they crave chewy cookies, flavored yogurt, double-chocolate ice cream. The first ingredient in the label may be sugar, but the second ingredient is fat.

Fats and Disease: What's the Connection?

Did you know that approximately 100 years ago, heart attacks were scarce in the US? In the early 1900's only about 3% of us died from heart disease. Today, nearly half of our population has some type of heart disease. More than one million people die annually in this country from heart attacks.

But in the early 1900s, people ate fresh, whole foods, including meat, butter and even lard! So why didn't they all die of heart attacks? The Food Giants have transformed God's natural fats into damaging fats, and they have convinced the American public to switch from butter to margarine and other processed oils.

Butter Is Better

Do you know butter is referenced nearly a dozen times in the Bible? Again, science proves the validity of the scriptures. One Medical Research Council survey published in *Nutrition Week*, showed that men eating butter ran half the risk of developing heart disease as those using margarine.[51]

Dr. Royal Lee, a dentist, inventor and nutritionist way ahead of his time, considered butter one of the best foods we could eat. He taught that fats were vital for a healthy immune and endocrine system and that butter is better than margarine even though it is higher in cholesterol. You can safely use butter in small amounts. A good replacement for margarine can be made by mixing equal amounts of warm butter with an unrefined oil like extra virgin olive oil. It's not only delicious, but it's also quite spreadable.

What Is a Trans Fat?

Trans fats are fats that have been altered or damaged by high heat. The fats God made are called natural or cis fatty acids. Trans fats are not found anywhere naturally, but are the result of a man-made process where a vegetable oil is hydrogenated by adding hydrogen molecules so what would normally be a liquid oil now becomes solid at room temperature. A good example of this is margarine. This process also makes vegetable oils saturated.

Studies have shown that margarine actually coats the stomach wall, rendering foods indigestible. (This doesn't even sound health sustaining. Don't you think they should put this on the label?) Margarine, shortening, and spread blends are all hydrogenated.

These trans-fatty acids not only raise the bad LDL cholesterol level, just like saturated fat, but they also lower the good HDL cholesterol. They hinder your body's ability to use the fat-soluble vitamins, they add to the load of our already overworked liver, and they even cause a greater essential fatty acid deficiency.

Foods Which Contain Trans Fats

· Shortening	· Potato chips	· Commercial peanut butter
· Taco shells	· Margarine	· Commercial vegetable oils
· Deep fried foods	· Snack foods	· Commercial mayonnaise
· Most donuts	· Salad dressings	· Commercial baked goods
· Corn chips		

Label reading is tricky. Just because the label says "all vegetable" oil does not mean it's healthy. It depends on what oil they used and whether or not it's been hydrogenated. Most restaurants use either processed heat-treated vegetable oils, or hydrogenated vegetable margarines, or both, although there is a healthy trend towards using real butter.

The Best Oil

Thou shalt have olive trees throughout all thy coasts.... Deuteronomy 28:40.

One of the most popular Bible foods is olive oil. Olive oil has been a staple for 5,000 years. The Greek Island of Crete, which has the highest olive oil consumption in the world has the lowest mortality rate due to cardiovascular disease. Most populations who use olive oil have a much lower incidence of heart disease and strokes.

Olive oil can help lower blood pressure and blood sugar, and can help reduce cholesterol and triglyceride levels while increasing HDL. Olive oil also improves digestion and helps to prevent gallstone formation.

Americans are eating high-fat foods, but are virtually fat deficient and deficient in vitamins A and E. Olive oil is high in vitamin E and may even improve the health of diabetics because olive oil helps regulate blood sugar levels.

There are three types of olive oil: Extra-virgin, virgin, and pure. Extra-virgin means the oil was pressed without further refinement. I prefer this type, but the flavor is strong. Virgin olive oil is filtered and has a milder taste than extra-virgin. Pure olive oil is a blend of refined olive oil and extra virgin or virgin olive oil. All of these unrefined oils are found in most health food stores. However, some "pure"and "light" olive oils found in the supermarket may be processed with the use of solvents so when buying these oils in the supermarket, I recommend buying the least refined ones (extra-virgin).

While it's not considered a saturated fat, olive oil does tend to become solid when put in the refrigerator. Don't worry. Just run it under hot tap water for a minute to "thaw" it out. (Don't zap it in the microwave! You'll make it a trans or damaged fat.)

Another Great Fat

Since 1971, our government has spent $30 billion on the War on Cancer, and yet cancers are far more common today than twenty years ago. But God knew that different fats have different effects on tumor growths. A type of fat called Omega 3 fatty acids have been clinically proven to reduce tumor growth. Proverbs 31:13 mentions flaxseeds, a great source of Omega 3 fat that has many health benefits.

Dr. Max Gerson, famous cancer researcher of the Gerson Institute in Mexico, used flaxseed oil for lowering cholesterol and dissolving tumors. Dr. Johanna Budwig also used flaxseed oil for successfully treating cancer and diabetes.

There is growing evidence that Omega 3 fatty acids from flaxseeds can improve behavior in children, boost their IQ, and improve their immune system.

Good, Fatty Fish

The Israelites were great fish eaters (Matt. 14:17-21; John 21:9-12) and probably ate fish daily.

Fish is a healthy alternative to beef. Some of the latest research in heart disease has been done using salmon. The Greenland Eskimos, for example, eat a diet rich in cold-water salmon, yet they have very little heart disease.

Cold-water fish are high in Omega-3 fat that has proven to reduce the risk of heart disease and high blood pressure, prevent blood clots, boost the immune system, protect against cancer and feed the brain. There are many benefits of essential fats. They:

- Carry and store fat-soluble vitamins A, D, E, and K (for skin and blood clotting).
- Are necessary to make healthy hair, skin, and nails.
- Are vital for a healthy immune system.
- Are required to build hormones and assist in the treatment and prevention of PMS and other hormonal problems.
- Are an excellent source of energy.
- Help you handle stress better.
- Reduce food cravings and help you feel satisfied.
- Can lower triglycerides.
- Reduce tendency to form blood clots in arteries.
- Decrease total cholesterol and LDL.

Here are good cold-water fish:

· Salmon	· Halibut	· Trout
· Perch	· Mackerel	· Tuna
· Haddock	· Red snapper	

Obviously, deep fried anything is out, since frying leads to free radical damage, which is linked to cancer. Shellfish are higher in cholesterol and have a poor filtration system which means they can retain toxins. From a nutritional standpoint, these scavengers are higher in saturated fats, so they are not healthy. (Even our fishing waters can be polluted. Problems with DDT, a carcinogen, and PCB's are rampant. When possible, look for safe sources of fish.)

We Need Some Protein

Surprisingly, many of my female clients, in their attempts to eat healthier, don't get enough protein. We need good quality protein daily. Proteins build muscle, bone, cartilage, and skin. They help make new hair and nails, replace worn cells, and regulate the body's functions and fluids. And having adequate protein also boosts your metabolism.

Protein Sources

Animal foods such as dairy, milk, meat, and eggs provide all of the essential amino acids and make a complete protein and are great sources of iron, B12 and other B vitamins.

Beans are a wonderful source of both fiber and protein. They are excellent for weight loss since they are high in protein, contain no fat, and their high-fiber content makes them low on the glycemic index. As a protein source, they complement whole grains, which means that beans and grains combined in a whole-foods diet make a complete protein equal to that of animal meat protein.

While Americans are most familiar with beans in chili and Mexican food, the most popular legume in the Bible was lentils (Gen. 25:34). Lentils are the easiest to cook and digest.

Soybeans are high in vitamins and protein, and are low in calories, carbohydrates, and fats. Soybeans are the highest in protein of all the beans.

Research shows that soy protein may help reduce the risk of breast cancer, osteoporosis, and post-menopausal symptoms in women. Additionally, a regular intake of soy protein may result in a reduction of coronary heart disease and a decrease in LDL cholesterol.

However, recent research shows that soy can be an allergen, and that most soy products are heavily sprayed with pesticides. Additionally, people can get too much soy, which can cause abnormal hormone levels in both males and females. Because of this, there is a concern about giving soy milk to young children. Be moderate with soy milk and only use natural soy foods such as tempeh and tofu. Take digestive enzymes or Beano for help in digesting beans and soy products.

How Did People Eat in Bible Days?

In Bible days, meat was eaten as part of celebrations, a few times a month, as reflected in the Mediterranean Food Pyramid. The most popular meats mentioned in the Bible were beef, lamb, goat and venison. Bible meats were "organically" grown in the sense that there was no need to use antibiotics; their animals were well nourished which kept their immune systems strong. God had specific instructions for raising, killing, and preparing meat, which protected man from diseases. There were no mad cows back then; they were all pretty happy!

Today, the Food Giants use antibiotics and hormones to make the animals fatter and grow faster. However, high hormone levels in meat and even dairy products have been linked to female problems in American woman. Some people believe that eating processed animal foods causes menstruation at an earlier age which increases the risk of developing cervical or breast cancer.

Eggs are another Biblical food mentioned in various scriptures and are recommended a few times a week in the Mediterranean diet. But eggs, like butter have also gotten a bad wrap by the Food Giants. Eggs themselves don't raise cholesterol. The myth that they do was based on one single, faulty study done years ago with powdered, processed eggs. It was the processing that raised the cholesterol, not the eggs. The lecithin and choline in the yolk of eggs can actually lower cholesterol.

The milk drank in Bible days was different than the milk we drink today, which is processed by the Food Giants.

Pasteurizing promotes shelf life, not our life. Raw milk can be refrigerated and stays fresh for about a week. Pasteurized milk will last two weeks, but it won't go sour, it will rot. Pasteurizing kills the natural bacteria, which is nature's way to preserve milk. Calves can't live on pasteurized milk!

In his book, *Why Christians Get Sick,* George Malkmus explains that milk is pasteurized when it's heated to at least 160 degrees to kill bacteria, which destroys almost the total nutritional value of the milk. Then it is homogenized so that the cream won't rise to the top, and finally coal tar derived vitamins are added in an attempt to replace some of the natural vitamins removed in processing. He says that most people are unaware that pasteurization renders the calcium unusable by the body because heat changes the organic calcium found in raw milk to an inorganic form. The body can only utilize organic minerals.[52] We are the greatest milk-drinking nation, yet we also have the highest rates of osteoporosis, a disease linked to calcium metabolism.

Today's milk is from unhealthy cows, fattened with hormones and drugged with antibiotics and then pasteurized —it's no wonder millions of people can't digest it!

Goat's milk was the most common milk used in Bible days. Since goat's milk is so close to mother's milk, and easy to digest, I recommend that mothers who can't breastfeed use goat's milk. The best milk for infants is breast milk, and studies have shown that breastfed babies have stronger immune function and less allergies. Processed formulas can't compare to breast milk and goat's milk for healthy babies.

In Biblical times, milk was consumed in the form of yogurt, feta cheese, cottage cheese or butter, and only in small quantities. These foods were popular probably because fermenting them was a way of keeping them longer, since it kept them from spoiling quickly. These foods are packed with calcium and magnesium and since they are pre-digested, they are easier for most people to digest. They were commonly made from sheep and goats.

Yogurt, when properly fermented, contains Lactobacillus acidophilus and other healthy bacterias. The bacteria in yogurt is a friendly, or good bacteria often called a probiotic. Yogurt restores good bacteria that is destroyed by antibiotics, and is highly recommended following any treatment with antibiotics to replenish this good bacteria. However, forget the coffee, mocha, cappachino, and sugar-sweetened yogurts!

There are dozens of references to nuts and seeds in the Bible, and traditional cultures eat them in a variety of ways. The best nuts are raw (not roasted, toasted, and dead!) which make a wonderful snack, provided you only eat a handful at a time.

Nuts are great sources of fiber, protein, vitamins, minerals, and "healthy" fats. Nuts are high in cancer-fighting antioxidants. Brazil nuts are especially high in selenium, a great antioxidant. Almonds are high in vitamin E, magnesium, folic acid, and calcium. Walnuts are high in Omega 3 fats. Sesame seeds are a good source of calcium. Sunflower seeds have protein, calcium, iron, B vitamins and good fats. Pumpkin seeds, known for their zinc are great for prostate health.

Let's see how much God cares about what you eat today.

PART THREE

God Cares About What You Eat

And God said, Behold, I have given you every herb bearing seed, which is upon the face of all the earth, and every tree, in the which is the fruit of a tree yielding seed; to you it shall be for meat.

Genesis 1:29

Chapter Eight

Dietary Guidelines From God

Switching from processed foods to more natural foods took some adjustment for me. When I first started to learn how to cook, it was a religious experience—everything I made was either a sacrifice or a burnt offering!

Have you been confused as to what in the world we are supposed to eat and why? Hey, you're certainly not alone. While we have been bombarded with thousands of foods made by the Food Giants, we have to remember who made everything—God. If you ever doubt that God was the original creator of all things, re-read and meditate on Job 38:4 to 39 *(NAS)*:

Where were you when I laid the foundation of the earth? After God asked Job this question, He explained the intricate details of His creation. Read it; it's pretty amazing stuff.

In this chapter, we'll hit the highlights of the significant scriptures in which He clearly gives us His Biblical nutritional guidelines in the Old Testament.

In the Beginning

Right after God created the heavens, earth, sky, light and darkness, God created plants "which yield seed" (Gen. 1:11-12). This included whole grains, fruits, vegetables, legumes, nuts, seeds and herbs, all foods similar to the simple natural diet eaten by the long-lived cultures mentioned earlier in this book. Next God created "every living creature that moves" but not necessarily for food (verses 21, 24). God created the food and animals first and then the man (27). God intended man to eat plants and fruits (29), and animals to eat herbs (30).

What a Miracle

God created the first man from the dust of the earth (Gen.2:7). He just picked up some dirt and all of a sudden—boom—here's a man! He put him in the Garden of Eating—oops, I mean Eden. This is significant because God was telling us that He made man from this rich earth; the very substance that He wants us to grow food in, is factory specified to nourish our bodies! Man could now be nourished by the vitamins and minerals in the vegetation and trees planted in the soil that God made.

Gen. 2:15 says that then God took the man and put him in the Garden of Eden to cultivate and keep it. Growing food to eat was (and still is!) an important job.

Soil Is Precious to God

An interesting sidenote regarding the soil is found in Leviticus 25:1-6. The Lord told Moses they should farm for six years, but during the seventh year the land should have a rest — for an entire year. Many farmers believe that God had a rotation plan in Leviticus to insure soil rich in nutrients which would feed man perfectly. Unfortunately, our U.S. soils are seriously deficient of vital minerals, which is why today we need to supplement our diets. (For more information on our soils and nutrient deficiencies, see my book, *Why Do I Need Whole-Food Supplements?* listed at the end of this book.)

In Genesis 2:16-17, God put down his first commandment regarding food which was not to eat of the tree of the knowledge of good and evil. You know the story. In chapter 3, Eve was deceived, and she and Adam ate the wrong fruit. This must have been some fruit to attract them from the lucious, incredible fruit in the Garden! But God's guidelines for Eve were for her protection as they are for us today.

Just as Eve was deceived in the Garden, man is equally deceived today if he believes he has the wisdom to improve upon the food that God made. Although processed foods manufactured by the Food Giants may look like the real thing, they aren't. Today, genetically engineered foods look like the original food, but time will tell their true impact on humans.

In Genesis 3:18 God told Adam he would now eat the "herb" of the field which is also translated the "plants" of the field which were originally meant for the animals. (See Ps. 104:14). Adam went from the garden to the field; now Adam became a farmer and not just a caretaker. As long as we exist, we will be able to plant seeds and watch them grow (Gen. 8:22).

Was Sixty Middle Aged Then?

We see from chapter 5 that men lived long lives—some between the ages of 700 to 900 years old. Hard to imagine and even harder to achieve! But Genesis 6:3 says that man's years would be 120. From a nutritional standpoint, living 120 years is possible. In Dr. Reginald Cherry's book, *The Bible Cure,* he quoted research done in the early fifties at the University of California in San Francisco that all human cells were able to reproduce themselves about fifty cell divisions, which placed the human life at about one hundred twenty years.[53]

Some people say they wouldn't want to live that long, but they might if they were still healthy, active and serving the Lord!

It's Okay to Eat Meat

Finally in Genesis 9:3 God said to Noah after the Flood, *Every moving thing that liveth shall be meat (food) for you...* But man was not supposed to eat meat with the blood still in it. This is still good advice since raw blood is the carrier of disease.

Noah most likely only ate clean meat on the ark. An interesting note is that Noah was 600 years old (Gen. 7:6) when God had him load the ark, so it appears that prior to that time, he may have lived on a vegetarian diet. While people still debate whether man was supposed to eat meat or not, it's interesting that Noah lived to be 950 years old, 350 more years after the flood, with the option of meat in his diet. (We'll look more at the issue later in this chapter and the next chapter.)

Hello Down There!

So far we see God's provision and two indications of His communication with both Adam and Noah regarding food. That God cares about whether we obey Him or not is clearly shown

again in Exodus 16:4 *(AMP)*: *Then said the Lord unto Moses,...
I will rain bread from heaven for you... that I may prove them,
whether they will walk in My Law or no.* This had to be relating
to diet, because the context of this chapter is their experience
with getting "manna," or bread-like wafers which were rained
from heaven. They ate manna for 40 years. God wanted them
to trust Him as their provider so much that He even had them
save a portion of it in a pot for future generations to see.

Hey, I'll Keep You Well!

In Exodus 15:26, right before He rained manna from heaven,
He said, "If you will obey me and my laws... you won't get
sick!" (my paraphrase). There was a condition to the promise
that they obeyed His laws. Let's look at an example that shows
us that He was serious about this.

Selfish, Whiny Babies?

The Israelites had the same trouble with their appetites then
as we do today. In Numbers 11:4-5, the Israelites complained
saying they remembered and wanted the fish, cucumbers,
melons, garlic, onions and leeks they ate in Egypt. God was so
angry with them that He told them He would give them flesh, so
much so that it would be for a whole month and it would come
out of their nostrils and be disgusting for them because they
despised the Lord and complained! Numbers 11:33, 34 says:

And while the flesh (meat) *was yet between their teeth, ...the
wrath of the Lord was kindled against the people, and the Lord
smote the people with a very great plague.* Yuck! He must have
been very mad!

The place was called "Kibroth-hattaavah" because they
buried the people there whose physical appetite caused them to
sin. God wanted their future generations to remember this.

But God Is a Good God!

We have to remember that God is a good God, full of mercy
and love (Ps. 103:17), but He hates sin and rebellion. Psalm
107:20 says, *He delivered them from their destruction.* The

Israelites, like Eve, Esau, Eli and others lusted after food which caused their own destruction. God was trying to save them from themselves by supplying them with manna. He didn't want them to become like the rest of the world.

Let's Get to God's Guidelines

Up until now we've looked at creation, attitude and obedience. Let's go specifically to Leviticus and Deuteronomy, books of the Pentateuch that all Jewish believers were required to know.

Leviticus 11 and Deuteronomy 14 were written for the Israelites to teach them the difference between clean and unclean foods. And to make matters very clear, their physical structure indicated whether they were clean or not.

One type of unclean animal refers to scavenger-type birds and fish which are defined as "any animal that eats refuse and decaying organic matter." These animals ate dead carcasses of other animals. Talk about a junk food diet!

Clean and Unclean Animals

Clean fish were identified as fish with both fins and scales (salmon, perch, tuna and mackerel). Unclean fish do not have fins and scales (shellfish, lobster, crab, oysters, and shrimp).

Clean birds were non-scavenger birds, and birds that fly as opposed to walking or creeping (such as turtledoves, pigeons, turkey and chicken). Unclean birds are birds of prey (vulture, eagle, raven and bat) and birds that creep or walk and do not fly (ostrich and stork).

Clean fish with fins and scales have a filtration system like our sweat glands, while shellfish don't have a filtration system and are mostly scavengers. The nutritional significance is that a filtration system insures that the fish don't easily store toxins from the ocean, as the scavengers do. Salmon, mackerel, halibut and tuna are rich in the natural Omega 3 fatty acids, all proven to prevent heart disease, cancer and diabetes. Scavengers and shellfish, on the other hand, raise the risk of heart disease due to their high cholesterol content.

Clean beasts have a divided hoof and chew the cud, which indicates more than one stomach, and are grass-eating animals (sheep, ox, deer and cow). Unclean animals can have a divided hoof but not chew the cud, or not have a divided hoof, and chew the cud, but they don't have both which is how God identified them (camel and horse). Animals which don't chew the cud only have one stomach. This means the food they chew is not well digested.

Pigs especially have poor elimination systems (no sweat glands), thus the (undigested) material they eat is often not easily removed from their flesh. They are scavengers that love to feed on dead cattle and horses, they often contain parasites and are a high source of cholesterol. I gave up eating pork when I was in my twenties years before I even heard of Leviticus 11. I had read numerous books on health and nutrition and discovered that pork is high in fat and is a high risk food in terms of danger of disease and tapeworms. Since that time, I've seen the blood samples of hundreds of people who eat pork, and it's generally swarming with unwanted bacteria. No thanks!

Other unclean beasts included rabbits and other rodents. These chapters also describe clean and unclean insects; and clean and unclean animals with paws and that creep. (I bet even Fear Factor contestants wouldn't eat creepy crocodiles and lizards!)

The Connection Between Holiness and Food

As we look at these scriptures, it's important to see how they fit into the big picture. Leviticus 10:10 *(NAS)* precedes chapter 11 with, *And so as to make a distinction between the holy and the profane* (unholy), *and between the unclean and the clean.*

Leviticus 11:45-47:

> *For I am the Lord...ye shall therefore be holy, for I am holy. This is the law of the beasts* (animals) *and of the foul* (birds) *and of every living creature that moveth in the waters, or and of every creature that creepeth upon the earth: To make a difference* (distinction) *between the unclean and the clean, and between the beast* (animal) *that may be eaten and the beast* (animal) *that may not be eaten.*

Then Deuteronomy 14:2-3 (*NIV*) says: *For you are a holy people holy to the Lord your God. Out of all the peoples on the face of the earth, the Lord has chosen you to be His treasured possession. Do not eat any detestable thing.*

Just Be Holy

In Leviticus 11, He summarizes the chapter with an admonition to be holy, and in Deut. 14, He began the chapter about being holy.

In other words, God himself, clearly linked being holy with following His Dietary Law.

Remember the first chapter of Daniel, where he chose not to defile himself with food and he chose a diet of grains, beans, vegetables nuts and seeds? He also refused the king's food, which could have included unclean foods. I believe Daniel ate this way as a lifestyle, not as a temporary fast as some have suggested, because the long-lived people have survived well on this way of eating.

Some New Testament scriptures also link cleansing of the physical temple with being holy before God.

2 Cor. 7:1 *Let us cleanse ourselves from all filthiness of the flesh* (body) *and spirit.*

1 Cor. 6:19, 20 reminds us our bodies are His; I Thes, 4:3 says we are still a consecrated people; Rom 12:1, 2 says we are to offer ourselves as sacrifices and be not conformed to the world (and it's food).

Our salvation no longer depends on our diet, but there is a definite link between our diet and our holiness before the Lord individually. For example, it's much easier for me to be obedient to the Lord in prayer and fasting, when I have been eating lighter and wholesome foods. Unclean foods cause a toxic bloodstream; it's really hard to fast when your blood is toxic!

What Are We Redeemed From?

How does this information affect us today? Let's begin by defining the Laws of the Old Testament.

Most people know there is a Moral Law consisting of the Ten Commandments in Exodus 20:1-17.

There was a Civil Law that God gave Israel to govern with (Matt. 22:21). And there were definitely Sanitation Laws (Leviticus 14:8, 9) which are practices used today by medical science. The Bible was thousands of years ahead of medical science in practices of sanitation.

Throughout the scripture, there is an emphasis on cleanliness. Was God a neat freak? You bet!

In Sharon Broer's book, she tells moms to help their children avoid food-borne illnesses by enforcing hand-washing with your children. She tells the story of a freshman named Annie who experimented, going through the entire day without washing her hands. She set up four petri dishes. She compared samples collected from her unwashed hands, with her hands rinsed under cold water, and her hands washed with soap and water, and finally her hands scrubbed with an antiseptic soap. There were hundreds of thousands of colonies of bacteria in the first two dishes. So rinsing with water didn't help. In dishes three and four, where the hands were cleaned, there were nearly no microbes.[54]

There also was a Ceremonial Law which had to do with the sacrifices. When Jesus died on the cross, He fulfilled the Ceremonial law in Romans 10:4: *Christ is the end of the law for the righteous.* We no longer need bulls and goats to offer for our sins; Jesus' blood has redeemed us once and for all.

We still should obey the Civil and Sanitation Law and we are still accountable for the Moral Law with the Ten Commandments. Jesus clearly fulfilled the Ceremonial Law. Then what about the Dietary Law? Are we accountable for it?

Same Law, Different Reasons

Yes! God gave the principles of how the Dietary Law worked, and it's still applicable today. However, we have a different reason than the Jews did for following the Dietary Law. They could not eat unclean foods because it affected their righteousness before God. Whether we eat pork or not does not affect our salvation, but it does affect our health. Following the law isn't required to get to Heaven, but not following it will get us there sooner!

Do Lobsters Have Fins?

But what about the animals listed in the Old Testament as clean and unclean? Did Jesus' dying on the cross mean that pigs have sweat glands now or lobsters now have fins? No, pigs, lobsters, and people are all the same today as they were then. A scavenger back then is still a scavenger today, and if we eat them today, we will be exposed to the same disease today as back then.

I believe you are free to eat what you want (I Cor. 6:12, 10:23). However, the Bible also says to know the truth and it will make you free (John 8:32), we perish for lack of knowledge (Hosea 4:6), and that knowledge brings deliverance.

How To Live a Longer Life

When I began to understand the Dietary Laws from the scriptures, I realized that I had been following them unconsciously all these years and I was reaping the results. The Bible promises in Proverbs 3:1, 2: *Forget not my law, but let thine heart keep my commandments. For length of days and long life and peace shall they add to thee.* I believe this means **all** of His commandments—His Dietary and Health Laws included, because when we break these laws listed above, we become sick.

An Inside Job

There's another scripture that the Lord gave me when I was studying this and it's Jeremiah 31:33, *I will put my law in their inward parts, and write it in their hearts; and will be their God, and they shall be my people.* (Cross references are Ps. 37:31, 40:8, 32:40, and Heb. 8:10.)

In other words, when God made us, He established what foods would and wouldn't work to keep us healthy and wrote it in our inward parts (our cells and internal organs) and when we obey His laws, (all, including Dietary Laws) we are healthy which leads to long life; (healthy cells and organs) and when we don't, we fall into sickness and death.

We all know what we should eat. Even small children who come into my office with their parents know when they have eaten too much sugar and candy! Long-lived cultures who are not necessarily even born again live long just by (accidentally) following His Dietary Laws.

Let's Review

Before we look at how the New Testament looks at the Dietary Laws, let's review what they were and were not.

1. The original Dietary Laws did not forbid meat eating in general, but rather certain types of meat that were, for health reasons, unsafe to eat on a regular basis.

2. Included in the Dietary Law were distinctions between clean and unclean fish, poultry, insects, and animals.

3. The Dietary Law didn't forbid any grains, nuts, beans, seeds, fruits or vegetables whatsoever. All were considered clean.

4. The Dietary Law forbade the drinking of the blood of an animal (Lev. 7:26-27, 17:10-14, Deut. 12:23-25) (I encourage my clients not to eat raw meat; blood carries the toxins and larvae of worms.)

5. The Dietary Law forbade eating the fat around the organs of the ox, sheep or goat (Lev. 3:17, 7:23) which God considered harmful and is still considered to cause heart disease.

6. The Ceremonial Law followed the guidelines of the Dietary Law because these sacrifices were: Lambs, goats, rams, calves, bulls, pigeons and turtledoves, all clean foods which the Israelites were allowed to eat.

7. They were not to take wine or strong drink (Lev. 10:9-11).

By the way, junk foods, as we know them were not part of the Dietary Law.

The Israelites probably ate milk, cheese, breads, fruits, vegetables, nuts and seeds and clean meat. They didn't drink the blood of animals, eat their fat or take strong drink. They probably lived on a diet very similar to the long-lived cultures, and ate more fish than meat and dairy. As long as they obeyed the Dietary Law, they were doing their part physically to receive God's blessing of health and long life.

So by now you might be wondering about those confusing verses about the "law" in the New Testament. Read on.

Chapter Nine

Did Jesus Eat Pork?

Wouldn't it have been nice if the Bible would have included an entire chapter on the exercise and eating habits of Jesus? We could just read the summary at the end of the chapter and know for sure how He lived.

The chapter would have gone something like this... "For breakfast, Jesus ate a delicious, Asparagus Omelette (the egg of clean animals) and Barley Bread. After walking around the towns and villages ministering to people for hours, he met with the disciples at Peter's house for lunch. They all sat down to some Grilled Salmon with Dill Sauce and homemade Whole Wheat Foccachia Bread with Garlic." (Yummm!) And on it would go, describing everything He did and ate.

Who Can We Ask?

But there is no chapter like this, so we must read between the lines and study the culture of the day. The best people to ask about longevity are the people who are living long, healthy lives eating traditional Bible foods.

Where are these people who live to be 100 years old in vigorous health? In her book, *Will Bible Foods Prevent Cancer?,* journalist Mary June Parks reported one man in Vilcabamba, Ecuador was 169 years old when he died. He was married to one woman for 102 years. (You know he had to be in good health!) She also said that the Hunzas died without ever suffering from a confining illness. This means they had no heart disease, cancer or diabetes! They exercised vigorously tending their organically grown crops. They had a balance of pure air, clean water, nutritious foods and exercise. She called their diet "Bible foods in the most literal sense."[55]

But many Christians are confused about the Dietary Law, Jesus' diet, and the seven frequently misunderstood references in the New Testament. Let's look at them.

All Meats Are Clean

Many people quote Mark 7:18-19 (*Weymouth*) saying that Jesus purged all meats so all meat is clean now. We can eat anything we want. We don't have to follow the Dietary Law.

> *Do you not understand that anything whatever that enters a man from outside cannot make him unclean, because it does not go into his heart, but into his stomach...By these words Jesus pronounced all kinds of food clean.*

The *Amplified Version* sheds more light on this verse: *Thus He was making and declaring all foods (ceremonially) clean (that is, abolishing the ceremonial distinctions of the Levitical Law.).* Foods that are ceremonially unclean refers to food that had been offered to idols. So what this verse really is saying is all foods that have been sacrificed to idols are clean.

There is no indication that God had gone against what He said in the Old Testament. Malachi 3:6 says that God never changes. But what we need to know is that when Paul was discussing food here, he was only referring to the clean meats in the Dietary Law since unclean meat was never considered by a practicing Jew, like Paul, to be "food."

Verse 18 is often quoted as saying that it doesn't matter what we eat any more. *The New King James Version* says: *Whatever enters a man from outside cannot defile him.* In this context, Jesus was addressing what's in the heart, not what's in the body.

Your Dinner Is Served

People often quote Luke 10:8, *Eat such things as are set before you* saying that God has given them permission to eat anything set in front of you. Hey, I'll have a pizza and a coke!

Here's my problem with that interpretation. Why would God write almost two full chapters on Dietary Laws, and over 900 references on specific foods and even design animals so as to discern clean from the unclean and then tell you to eat whatever is in front of you? If someone served you a cardboard box, would you eat it? (Some of the cereals I've had taste like cardboard boxes, but that's beside the point. We have to rightly divide the Word!)

The thing to remember about this verse is that Jesus was ministering to the Jews, who already knew the Dietary Laws. In fact, one of the reasons why the New Testament doesn't dwell on the issue of food is that they were all practicing Jews, including Jesus, and they all ate kosher food. We know that by reading the New Testament. The scripture deals with not being concerned with whether these clean foods had been offered to strange gods.

Of Sheets and Men

Many people consider Acts 10:13-15, the vision of Peter as evidence that clean and unclean distinctions were abolished. Peter knew what was clean and unclean and closely followed these laws (Acts 10:14). Verse 28 in the *Williams* translation says, *God has taught me not to call any man vulgar or ceremonially unclean....* God himself told Peter that he should not call any **man** unclean. He was referring to men, not food. If God were changing His Dietary Laws, He could have taken this opportunity and also clearly called food clean, but he didn't. He was making a point that the Jews were preaching to the Gentiles.

Sacrificial Offerings

Several verses in First Corinthians can be confusing until you understand what Paul was saying. First Corinthians 8:1-13 and 10:25-33 discuss food sacrificed to idols.

1 Cor. 8:4, 6, 7 The Simple English Bible:

You wrote me about eating meat which has been offered to false gods. We know that they really don't exist. There is only one true God. To us there is only one God—The Father. However, not everyone has this spiritual knowledge. Some people still have the habit of treating idols as though they were real when they eat such meat. Their conscience is weak; they feel that the food makes them unclean.

Verse 13: *Therefore, if meat causes my brother to sin, I will never eat meat.*

Eating foods offered to idols in the presence of a "weaker" brother might cause him to fall away from the faith. Again, Paul was referring to "clean" meat here. However, he was saying that he was willing to stop eating "clean" meat if it caused his brother to sin.

First Corinthians 10:23 in *The New English Bible* says it clearer:

> *We are free to do anything, you say. Yes, but is everything good for us? We are free to do anything, but does everything help the building of the community? Each of you must regard, not his own interests, but the other man's.*

What Paul isn't saying is, "Now we can do anything—lie, cheat, and steal." What Paul meant were the things allowed by God. Anything that was prohibited in the Word was forbidden.

Paul was saying they were free to eat whatever they wish—whether it was sacrificed or not. However, they were not to become a stumbling block to those with a weaker conscience who didn't believe in eating meat offered to idols.

Meat, Vegetables and the Law

Now in Romans 14:14: *There is nothing unclean of itself, but to him that esteemeth any thing to be unclean, to him it is unclean.* Paul is again saying here that foods that God declared clean cannot be made unclean when offered to idols.

The key point in this chapter is summed up well in Romans 14:3 *(Phillips Translation)*:

> *One man believes that he may eat anything, another man, without this strong conviction, is a vegetarian. The meat-eater should not despise the vegetarian, nor should the vegetarian condemn the meat-eater—they should reflect that God has accepted them both.*

One person believes he can eat all clean meats offered to idols and another person, fearful of being defiled by the idol, refuses to eat the meat (being a weaker Christian) and only eats vegetables.

Other key references in this chapter are verses 5 and 6 that refer to days and meats, referring to Jewish feasts and meats sacrificed to idols. Gentile Christians esteemed every day alike and had no problem with eating meats sacrificed to idols. Jewish Christians, however, still abstained from certain meats for fear that one of the meats might have been offered to idols.

Romans 14:17 says, *For the kingdom of God is not meat and drink; but righteousness, and peace, and joy in the Holy Ghost.* This means that being a Christian does not depend on your diet but your right standing before God.

How's Your Lifestyle?

Colossians 2:16 says: *Let no man therefore judge you in meat, or in drink, or in respect of an holyday, or of the new moon, or of the sabbath days.*

In this passage, Paul is telling the Colossians not to let anyone judge them concerning their salvation on the basis of what they ate or drank. Paul was really dealing with the same religious traditions of salvation through works. The issue here was not meat, but rather rituals. Verse 23 *(AMP)*: *These practices* (rituals) *are of no value in checking the indulgences of the flesh.*

God Bless My Candy Bar!

1 Timothy 4:4, 5: *For every creature of God is good and nothing to be refused, if it be received with thanksgiving: For it is sanctified by the word of God and prayer.*

This scripture is often quoted out of context, saying that God told us we could eat anything if we pray over it. Several keys here help accurately divide the Word. God created every creature, but not everything God created was to be eaten! This had to mean food created by God within God's laws: Clean meat, fish, dairy, vegetables, grains, fruits, nuts, and seeds.

Let's look at this phrase, "sanctified by the Word." What Word would that be? The only Word they had—the Old Testament Dietary Laws. In verse 3 it says, "those who know the truth" which points to Jews who knew the Dietary Law. Now look at the word, "sanctified," which means "set apart or sanctioned." What foods were set apart or sanctioned by God? The foods listed as clean in the Old Testament Dietary Laws. So the phrase the "Word and prayer" means foods authorized by the Bible.

Again, why would God call certain foods clean and unclean through the Bible and contradict Himself here? (Also, foods like candy bars are not created by God, but by the Food Giants and thus don't qualify as "good foods.")

Many Christians fool themselves by thinking they can, with prayer, "sanctify" food that God has definitely warned us against. Many Christians also unknowingly break health rules like the Dietary Laws and then pray for God to deliver them out of their own destruction. There are other natural laws written on our inward parts that Christians break as well, such as not eating or drinking too much—and then they also ask for prayer. Whether or not they admit it, they are still going against the Word of God. We need to do our part to live up to the promises.

The Same, Yesterday, Today, and Tomorrow

I believe God was serious about Christians not eating unclean foods and even today He wants us to study to show ourselves approved in areas like health and nutrition so we can "glorify God in our bodies."

Seventh Day Adventists, founded by Ellen G. White, have included in their teachings some strict rules on diet. For instance, they teach against using coffee, tea, tobacco, and alcoholic beverages. Also, they are taught not to eat pork. Statistics show that Adventists have less incidence of cancer, are healthier than most people, and as a group they live six years longer than the average American.

God wanted to protect His people through diet in the Old and New Testaments, and He still does today!

Let's now look at His powerful, protective foods with the purpose of healing.

Chapter Ten

Powerful, Protective Bible Foods

Sometimes it's hard to imagine how Jesus and His disciples ate. It's not like they could go down the street for a coffee at Starbucks or breakfast at McDonald's! They had to "catch" or "gather" all the food they ate. Boy, have times changed!

But the Israelites of the Bible were like us in many ways; they enjoyed eating and drinking. They cooked lentil soup; (Gen. 25:29); they ate apples and raisins as a snack (Solomon 2:5); and they baked bread (Ez. 4:9). But their foods were whole, natural foods. When they lusted for foods, they were for good foods. For example, in Numbers 11:4, 5 they wanted their meat, cucumbers, melons, garlic, onions and leeks. Their access to "junk" food was limited.

While there are a few diseases mentioned in the Bible, there is no mention of our major diseases today such as heart disease, strokes, high cholesterol or cancer. Their whole-foods diets protected them from many of what we call degenerative diseases.

People who lived during Bible days ate small amounts of meat, some fish, olive oil, and lots of fruits and vegetables. Legumes, like lentils, were a staple in their diet. Bible foods mentioned were high in fiber, and low in cholesterol. They had everything they needed in their food, and it was all balanced.

We don't have to be transported back to the Bible days to understand and appreciate how people ate. The food that people ate during Biblical times is close to the diet of Middle Eastern people who are in the Mediterranean area. Here is a short list of some foods they ate, which were and still are protective to our health. The number of Biblical references are also listed.

Almonds (5), apples (9), barley (97), bread (370), butter (10), cheese (3), corn (87), eggs (5), figs (57), fish (27), fruit (as food 9), grapes (50), honey (61), lamb (as food 3), lentils (4), milk (40), nuts (2), olives (35), oil (30), pulse (18), and wheat (52).

Other references are made to millet, dates, onions, garlic, leeks, pomegranates, herbs, salt, goat's milk, beef, venison, manna, and quail.

All of these foods have healing properties. God made food that would nourish, heal and lengthen your days. There is an obvious connection between disease and food. Eating right can prevent cancer, diabetes, heart disease, lower cholesterol, reduce high blood pressure, beat fatigue, boost your immune system, slow aging, get rid of PMS, and help your hair, skin and nails.

An interesting article in an old (January '73) issue of National Geographic by Alexander Leaf described the diets of other "long-lived" people living in the Georgian Soviet Socialist Republic in what was once called Russia, the Vilcabambas in Ecuador, and the Hunzas in Pakistani-controlled Kashmir. All three cultures ate simple, natural complex carbohydrates (whole grains, vegetable seeds, nuts and fruits, and very little animal foods.) They lived to be between 100-120 years old.

Traditional cultures today also eat many vegetable dishes which are excellent sources of vitamins and minerals, glucose and fiber. Leafy greens are loaded with rich sources of nutrients and enzymes. Traditional cultures eat fruits either fresh or dried and in season. Fruits are excellent sources of vitamins and minerals and are easily digested.

Even today, the more popular "weight loss diets" include fruits, vegetables, lean protein, and whole grain carbohydrates. Let's look at the link between Bible foods and science.

We Can't Outdo God!

The more science looks into natural whole foods, the more they see precise amounts and ratios of nutrients to produce synergistic harmony in the body. All of the essential elements needed are incredibly combined in whole foods. Health problems begin when we start to separate whole foods and then try to put them back together.

For example, if you isolate all the chemicals in a carrot, you might find a poisonous chemical. But we don't get sick eating a carrot because that element is combined quite naturally. These non-nutritive substances in plants are called phytochemicals or nutraceuticals. They are simply naturally occurring chemicals in plants which provide health benefits. To date, researchers have uncovered more than 100,000 phytochemicals.

For example, most people know about vitamins such as vitamin C. It's necessary for healthy tissue, especially skin, and a healthy immune system. Vitamin A is an anti-infection vitamin, and vitamin E with selenium, both antioxidants, are great protectors against pollution and pesticides. Together they make a mighty team. Antioxidants are found in nearly every natural food. For example, carrots, sweet potato, kale, butternut squash, pumpkin, cantaloupe, apricot, spinach and broccoli are rich in beta carotene, another antioxidant.

Why Eat Your Fruits and Vegetables?

People who eat more fruits and vegetables have stronger immune systems, fewer incidences of heart disease, arthritis, and high blood pressure.

Vegetables can slow the aging process. Jean Carper in her book, *Food—Your Miracle Medicine,* says that all fruits and vegetables are packed with antioxidants which defend our cells against attack by free radicals. Free radicals are the chemicals that damage and destroy cells, promoting aging and disease.[56]

Most of us eat salads for lunch only on occasion. We'll have a side order of cabbage slaw with a burger or a carrot salad at the deli. But salads are wonderful. The best part is they boost your metabolism. These foods have the fewest calories, highest nutrients, and antioxidants, or cancer-fighting chemicals.

Fruits and vegetables with the deepest colors, like red, orange and green, yield the highest antioxidant protection. Lutein, found in kale and broccoli, can protect the macula of the eye and a deficiency of lutein has been linked with macular degeneration.

Lycopene is a carotenoid like beta carotene which is also a powerful antioxidant against cancers. It's found in foods like tomatoes, red grapefruit, red peppers and watermelon.

Greens are high in chlorophyll. They are also high in iron, magnesium, calcium, manganese, vitamin C, potassium, vitamin A and some of the essential fatty acids. The darker the color, the higher the level of nutrients.

Red grapes contain flavonoids called polyphenols which strengthen capillary vessels and veins, helping repair varicose veins and bruising, for example. They can lower your risk of heart disease by inhibiting the formation of blood clots.

Try to eat 5-9 servings daily, of fruits vegetables. Choose from under-the-ground (potatoes, onions) and over-the-ground (leafy greens) vegetables. It's better to eat them fresh, or lightly steamed or sauteed. Frozen is preferred over canned. To preserve nutrients, buy produce as fresh as possible. Here are some references to Bible foods that we still eat today.

*Apples: Apples can lower blood cholesterol, blood pressure and the risk for cancer. High in soluble fiber, they help prevent sharp mood swings or stabilize blood-sugar levels; they contain a natural appetite suppressant, and are extremely high in potassium. (Joel 1:12, Song of Solomon 2:5)

*Almonds: Almonds are are high in vitamin E, magnesium, folic acid, and calcium. (Gen. 43:11)

*Barley: Barley is high in a special fiber that can lower the risk of heart disease by lowering LDL, the bad cholesterol. Barley contains some cancer-inhibiting elements. Barley is used mostly in soups. (Ruth 2:23, Ez. 4:9)

*Beans, whole: Beans are high in protein, fiber, and complex carbohydrates for energy. They help reduce LDL cholesterol and increase HDL cholesterol. Their fiber helps prevent colon cancer and regulate blood-sugar levels. (Ez. 4:9)

*Carob: Carob is a low-sugar, low-sodium, high-potassium and high-fiber food, often used as a replacement for chocolate in candy. (Matt. 3:4)

*Cheese, cottage cheese: Is a great source of protein, easier to digest than milk because it's predigested. (Gen. 18:8)

*Corn: Corn is the staple food of the Tarahumara Indians of Mexico who have almost no heart disease. (Ruth 2:14)

*Cucumbers: Cucumbers aid digestion, cleanse the bowels, and are helpful for breaking up cholesterol deposits. They help to promote healthy skin.(Nu. 11:5)

*Eggs: An excellent source of protein, the yolks are especially nutrient dense. They contain lecithin and choline, important nutrients for decreasing plaque formation. (Luke 11:12-113)

*Figs: Figs help prevent cancer and are anti-ulcer and anti-bacterial foods. They also reduce high-blood pressure. Figs are an excellent source of plant fiber for stabilizing blood-sugar levels. (Num. 13:23; Mark 11:112-13)

*Fish: Certain Omega 3 fish help lower blood cholesterol-levels, blood pressure and high triglycerides and prevent cancer and arthritis. Omega 3 oils are found in cold-water fish such as mackerel, salmon, and tuna. (John 21:9-13)

*Flaxseed: A rich source of Omega 3 fatty acids, flax is being used to help a variety of conditions including acne, allergies, arthritis, breast pain, diabetes, heart disease, learning disorders, menopause, obesity and stroke. (Prov. 31:13)

*Garlic: Garlic contains substances that help lower blood pressure, reduce cholesterol, and hinder the formation of blood clots. Garlic boosts the immune system and acts as a natural antibiotic. (Num. 11:5)

*Greens, bitter: Greens are high in vitamin A, high in fiber, low in calories, low in fat, and high in minerals. (Ex. 12:8)

*Grapes, raisins: Grapes are a good source of boron, and help ward off osteoporosis. Red grapes help prevent artery damage and heart attacks, and may lower blood pressure. (Deut. 23:24, Matt. 26:29; Song of Solomon 2:5)

*Grains, whole: Whole grains are rich in complex carbohydrates and are rich in fiber which can help reduce the risk of cancer. (Gen. 41:22)

*Honey: Raw honey contains bioflavonoids. (Ps. 81:16)

*Leeks: A long onion which looks like a large green onion. It's a blood purifier and aid for the liver. (Num. 11:5)

*Lentils: Lentils are a high-protein, high-fiber food. They are excellent food for diabetics and protect against high cholesterol. (Gen. 25:29, 34)

*Melons: Melons contain the antioxidant beta carotene and are high in fiber, potassium and vitamin C. (Nu. 11:5)

*Millet: Millet is a small gluten-free grain that makes a good substitute for rice. It has a nice light flavor. (Ez. 4:9)

*Pistachio: Most nuts contain anti-cancer and heart protective properties. They are full of antioxidants and monosaturated fat, which protect arteries from damage. (Gen. 43:11)

*Olive oil: Olive oil improves digestion, and helps decrease gallstone formation. Olive oil helps increase the good cholesterol, decrease bad cholesterol, and helps regulate blood-sugar levels. (Lev. 2:4; Lev. 8:8)

*Onions: Onions thin the blood, help lower cholesterol, help to prevent strokes and boost HDL, the good cholesterol. (Nu. 11:5)

*Wheat: Wheat is a whole-grain full of vitamins, minerals and bran. It's said to raise good cholesterol levels. Wheat has been the staple food of the Armenians, Greeks, Romans and Holy Land people for 4500 years. In the Biblical days, it was considered an important part of the diet. (Gen. 18:6 42!1 and 2, Gen 43:11; Ps. 81:16)

*Yogurt: Yogurt is high in protein and calcium and it contains certain bacteria which aid digestion, and help correct constipation. (Is. 7:15)

Mediterranean Meal Planning

The Mediterranean Diet included fresh fruits and vegetables, whole grains, beans, nuts, seeds, fresh fish and small amounts of animal protein.   My clients often ask me how they can incorporate these foods in their daily menus.

To help with this task, my assistants Anne and Carolyn helped me to go through my cookbook (*Why Can't I Lose Weight Cookbook*) and list these Mediterranean type foods with recipes and their page numbers. Here they are: (To order any of my books, see the last pages of this book.)

Breakfast Choices

Oatmeal would be the most popular choice for kids and adults. (Other grains include buckwheat, brown rice, and millet.) Fruit salad is nice in the summer: grapes, melon, apples and yogurt.

Elegant Eggs

Basic Omelette, 184

Poached Eggs, 186

Scrambled Eggs, 187

Great Grains

Almond Mushroom Rice, 191

Basic Brown Rice, 190

Oatmeal, 190

Old Fashioned Museli, 195

Snacks: figs, dates, raisins, nuts (pistachio, walnuts)

Lunch Choices

Some kind of Mediterranean Salad with Green lettuce or wild greens, carrots, onions, cucumbers, tomatoes, olive and Feta Cheese is nice. Make an olive oil/vinegar dressing with garlic or a Pita bread with meat or bean filling.

Super Salad Dressings

Avocado Dressing, 114

Basic Italian Vinaigrette Dressing, 112

Creamy Vinaigrette, 112

Lucious Salads

Almond Brown Rice Salad, 121

Carrot Raisin Salad, 122

Classic Mixed Green Salad, 116

Greek Salad, 117

Lucious Fruit Salad, 123

Taboulie Salad, 120

Dinner Choices

Some kind of cooked bean dish such as lentils with carrots and onions or baked beans go well with steamed vegetables. Grill some salmon, halibut or tuna baked with garlic and olive oil. Sweet potatoes accompany fish dishes nicely.

Vegetable Entrees

Garlic Roasted Potatoes, 128

Green Beans With Almonds and Baby White Onions, 129

Italian Mashed Potatoes, 128

Roasted Garlic, 127

Steamed Vegetables, 125

Lean Bean Dishes

Greek Lentils, 134

Honey Baked Beans, 136

Mediterranean Rollups, 143

Mediterranean Tacos, 137

Fabulous Fish and Meat

Dijon Perch, 179

Easy Baked or Grilled Fish, 179

Easy Salmon Bake, 180

Lemon Baked Halibut, 180

Desserts

Fruit Sorbet, 214

Banana Yogurt Dessert, 214

Brown Rice Pudding, 215

Pumpkin Pie, 218

Okay, let's move on to the more spiritual side of eating.

PART FOUR

Pick Up Your
Shield of Faith!

...having taken up the shield of faith,
with which ye will be able to quench
all the fiery darts of the evil one.
Ephesians 6:16
Worrell New Testament

Chapter Eleven

God's Part & Your Part

Jesus tells us in John 15:5 that He is the vine and we are the branches and that without Him we can do nothing. In this verse, He aptly shows us that we are designed to function **with** Him, not apart from Him. His life flows through us, as the life of the vine flows through to the branches. But sometimes it doesn't seem like it, does it?

My clients tell me they want to "eat like Jesus ate" but it's hard. They crave bad foods. They overeat. Or they can't change bad habits. Many of my clients have confided in me, that sometimes they get confused as to what they're supposed to do and what God is supposed to do.

Nothing Is Too Hard for God

What do you want God to do for you? How wonderful it would be if He would just take away your cravings or habits instantly. That used to be my prayer. If prayer burned calories, I would have been skinny, I prayed so much! I kept hoping that God would just "zap" me and I would be free. Of course, God could have done that.

God is so incredible, powerful and strong, He can deliver us with His baby finger. We've all heard of testimonies where people have been supernaturally delivered from drugs, smoking, drinking, and gluttony.

Most important, though, is to realize that when it comes to health and healing, God has already done some remarkable things! First, He sent Jesus to die on the cross for us. He redeemed us from our sinful nature. He created us in a mighty way; trillions of mechanisms perform all throughout our bodies day in and day out! What a powerful machine. When He designed us, He put the ability to heal in every cell!

Then on top of that, all food that God created is vital, full of live enzymes, packed with nutrition, phytochemicals, minerals, vitamins, and coenzymes. Eating a diet full of good protein, carbohydrates, vitamins, minerals, fat and water will nourish and keep our bodies well.

Then He gave us the *Holy Bible,* God's instruction manual. The Bible is one of the greatest history books ever written, and throughout the pages are hundreds of ideas of how to live a healthy life, including nutrition as we have seen in this book.

For example, as I mentioned earlier in this book, He told us how to grow healthy, organic soil; He warned us about the dangers of eating unclean foods, He told us not to eat too many sweets, and to not overprocess foods.

The only catch is that God doesn't want us living our lives, waiting for His touch. He wants us to do something. This sign I saw once in front of a church says it well: "Don't expect God to do through a miracle what He expects you to do through obedience."

God wants **us** to deal with our **body (flesh)** and train it (I Cor. 9:27). God doesn't ask us to obey His Word to punish us, but rather that we would enjoy life abundantly. So in this chapter we'll look at what God's part is and what our part is. In the following two chapters, we'll look at how to do our part.

God and Us

God is with you, helping and leading you to your victory.

For we are fellow workmen—joint promoters, laborers together—with and for God; you are God's garden and vineyard and field under cultivation; (you are) God's building.

1 Corinthians 3:9 *(AMP)*

Years ago when I went to Bible school, a teacher named Keith Moore told us about a prayer he prayed. He asked God to show him what it would be like without the Holy Spirit. Keith explained that all of a sudden, he couldn't play the piano, or when he was trying to study and teach classes, he couldn't think. There was no flow. He forgot things. I remember thinking what a remarkable thing that it was: God is such a part of us, we often don't know where He ends and where we begin!

But to be practical, sometimes it helps to just sit down and think about His part and ours. I've written a chart so we can distinguish between our part and God's part.

His Part	My Part
• He created food and the Dietary Laws	• Follow His ideas and examples regarding food
• God was the first organic farmer	• Eat foods as close to organic and as fresh as possible
• He draw us to Him	• Believe on Jesus and make Him Lord
• He illuminates our darkness	• We seek His wisdom through prayer and the Word
• He speaks to us	• We listen to Him
• He works His will in us	• We trust in Him
• He develops self control in us	• We expect self control
• He leads us to victory	• We follow Him
• He teaches us	• We gain knowledge of His Word on diet and exercise
• He delivers us from temptation	• We resist temptation
• He strengthens us	• We get strong in body, mind and spirit

It can be confusing unless we remember that we are a three-part being: Spirit, mind and body. Yes, we have a spirit, but the Bible shows us that we need to **do** something about our body (flesh).

Our mind actually makes the decision whether or not to give in to the flesh. If we just let ourselves, we will easily overeat, be lazy and give up. When **we choose** to exercise, or eat right, we are taking control of our body! Realize that while God doesn't do our exercise for us, He is with us to strengthen and encourage us to exercise.

God doesn't think our thoughts for us either. But He does tell us that if we study His Word, and meditate on His Words, then we will start to think like He does. For example, instead of wanting second helpings of food, we have to decide to eat in moderation. We have to "renew our minds" or remind ourselves that sugar isn't good for us; and then train our taste buds to enjoy the simple, wholesome food that God made, not food made by the Food Giants.

God **does** direct our steps, but we have to be doing something for Him to help us. I once heard this analogy that He leads us when we are moving, or doing something, not when we are standing still. Have you ever tried to turn a parked car? You can't. But after you get it moving, then you can turn it. That's how God works with us. We need to take some steps, and He will help us. There was a time when the only steps I took were from the kitchen to the TV with munchies in my hand. These were the wrong steps!

Instead of buying lots of high fat junk food, we will load our shopping carts with fresh fruits and vegetables. And with our minds, we can decide that it's an honor, privilege and responsibility to take care of our bodies, rather than a drudgery. All of these are important parts of working with God.

Find anointed teaching on diet and exercise, and pray for God's direction. Read some of my books, or find books written by some of the Christian health professionals I've mentioned. I also recommend materials by Christian authors Marty Copeland and Stormy Omartian.

God loves you. You are valuable to Him. He is always with you and He will never forsake you. He's just as committed to your being healthy as you are. He ready to work eternal changes inside you as you explore these together with His help. Phil. 2:13 *(AMP)* says it well:

> *(Not in your own strength) for it is God Who is all the while effectually at work in you—energizing and creating in you the power and desire—both to will and to work for His good pleasure and satisfaction and delight.*

So let's go on to the next chapter and look at some steps we can take to develop our self control and resist temptation.

Chapter Twelve

You Already Have Self Control!

Yes, it could have been easier for Jesus and the disciples to have self control than it is for us. After all, there were no magazines, no television commercials, fast food restaurants and no Godiva chocolate. They had to worry about more important issues of the day, like getting enough food to eat!

As a nutritionist, I often hear people say, "I know what I should do, but I don't have self control to do it."

As Christians, we don't usually smoke, drink or take drugs. No, we eat! We are tempted to do things like overeat, or eat the wrong foods, which can be equally harmful. But this temptation seems harmless at times, doesn't it? Yet today medical research has proven that wrong eating and overeating can literally lead to death by a heart attack, diabetes, cancer, or some other degenerative disease.

I know many people who start on a healthier diet. They eat healthy for a few months, and gradually begin to slack off. They begin drinking coffee and eating a donut for breakfast instead of their former healthier breakfast. Then they begin to eat high sugar foods again, thinking a little won't hurt. The next thing you know, they are completely off their healthy diet, and they have gained the ten pounds they lost.

Now they feel like they have no self control. I remember thinking that years ago when I thought that I would never overcome my bad eating habits.

How did it start? It all starts with a subtle lie. Lies are at the root of every compulsive behavior. After you get mentally hooked, you get physically hooked and the behavior is addictive or compulsive. Since the problem started with a lie, the way to get free is with the truth. I know this from experience because I was a compulsive overeater nineteen years ago, and I have been set free. Praise God!

I used to eat a lot when I weighed more pounds than I do now. In fact, I remember eating two or three bowls of breakfast cereal and then not even an hour later, I would be searching for a snack. I felt powerless to change, like there was something in me that made me eat. I was out of control. But today I am free from this compulsive behavior, and I believe it's possible for everyone to be free!

The Biggest Lie

Probably the greatest lie of the devil is that we have no choice and that we are victims of our circumstances, but this is not true. God gave us the ability to make choices. Deuteronomy 11:26 tells us that the Lord sets both blessings and curses before us, which implies that we get to choose which one we receive.

Like Adam, we have been given a free will. Adam was free to choose to eat from either tree. Daily we can choose to eat candy bars or green salads. We can exercise, or lay on the couch, watching exercise videos! We can be naturally or carnally minded and follow the things of the world (like fad diets), or we can be God minded and follow the wisdom of the Bible (good nutrition, self control, and exercise).

Two Cycles

Let's look at two different cycles. Let's call the first cycle, The World's Cycle and the second cycle, The Life Cycle.

The World's Cycle starts with stress: too much pressure, too much to do and too little time! So how do most people handle stress?

Americans run on coffee and diet soda! We eat junk food, fast food, and sugar-sweetened snack foods; anything to get us through the morning, through lunch, or just through the day. Stress generally leads to a bad diet. A bad diet usually leads to other bad habits such as poor sleep and an overall lack of interest in any type of movement or exercise. But there is a better way!

The Life Cycle

The Life Cycle starts with making the right choices by thinking the right thoughts, such as believing that you can change, and believing that God has designed health for you. In this cycle, you learn about eating right, fasting and exercise, and you then enjoy the benefits of good health that God has promised you! You can get back in The Life Cycle by learning about how to handle temptation.

Where Is My Self Control?

Everyone has self control. Galatians 5:22 in *The Simple English Bible* says: *But the product of the spirit produces: love, joy, peace, patience, kindness, goodness, faithfulness, gentleness and self control.*

We have all been given a measure of self control, but we have to exercise our will to use self control, like we exercise a muscle. The more we use it, the better we get.

Resist Temptation

Self control is also the ability to withstand temptation. When it comes to eating, the most important part is the moment of temptation. What will you do then? The idea is not to wait until the temptation comes, but to get strong before it comes.

Picture two fighters. One man attacks another man. Each time the one under attack withstands the attack. But if the man attacking is stronger, the one resisting will lose. If he gets strong, he can put the attacker down. It all depends on who is stronger.

In Christ, you are the stronger one! As a Christian, you have been given "spiritual" strength over the devil.

There will always be temptations. If this were not true, there would be no struggles! Everyone would exercise, eat right and be healthy (and I would be out of a job!) But there are temptations. So we have to exercise our self control to overcome temptation.

So let's look at four points about temptation.

Everyone Is Tempted With Something

1. Everyone is tempted, but we're so different in how we are tempted. I'm always amazed that some clients can resist sweets easily, while others struggle. As hard as it is to believe, there are actually people living on this planet, who do not like desserts. So don't think it strange that you can be tempted.

2. God doesn't tempt you. *Let no man say when he is tempted, I am tempted of God: for God cannot be tempted with evil, neither tempteth he any man.* James 1:13. Matthew 4 explains that the tempter is the devil. James further explains that every man is tempted when he is drawn away and enticed and baited by his own evil desire, lust and passion. (James 1:14-15 *AMP.*) People often think just the devil makes them do evil. But he uses our own lust to tempt us.

We cannot stop temptations from knocking at our door, but we can stop inviting them in and feeding them a full course dinner. Think about what tempts you. Maybe cigars or cigarettes provide no temptation to you, but a double chocolate fudge sundae, look out! Why? Because that's where your body is weak. If you had control over that area, you would not be tempted.

3. God won't let you be tempted beyond your ability to handle it. God is involved in your life. He knows everything about you. He knows your weakness for Godiva chocolate and Fritos corn chips! He knows that you will be tempted, but He makes sure that it's within your ability to resist. The resisting part is your job.

4. When the temptation comes, the way of escape comes along with it. It's the way out. Sometimes it might be that you are too busy to take time for a snack—when you weren't hungry anyway. Your mind was so busy with other things that you actually forgot about food. (That had to be "supernatural!")

Here are four tips for dealing with temptation.

How To Deal With Temptation

1. Pray. We need to pray **before** we enter into temptation. Prayer makes us stronger. When I first prayed for help, the Lord gave me 1 Cor. 10:13, so I asked Him for the way of escape.

Sometimes the whole day went by before I realize what He did for me. I didn't overeat, or I never made it to the lunch room to buy that candy bar. It didn't happen overnight. But the more I remembered to pray, the more I saw His answer to prayer.

2 Peter 2:9 says that He delivers the Godly from temptation. He knows what it was like to be tempted (Heb 2:18) so He can help you. When you pray, ask for the answer to your food problem, not just the problem with your weight.

2. Plan. Prov. 5:1-2 says to get wisdom. Gaining wisdom is part of proper planning and finding the answer to temptation.

When you are actually at the restaurant is not the time to start thinking about how to cope! Standing in the middle of the fiery darts is no time to start looking for the faith shield! It's much easier to resist an opponent if you know he's coming and are ready for him than if he catches you off guard.

a. Eliminate foods you don't want to eat. Create an environment conducive to health. If you only have fruit around, that's all you will eat. Throw out the M&Ms!

b. Plan your week's menus. Know what you will eat for breakfast, lunch and dinner and you won't be tempted by vending machines. If you don't plan it, you won't eat it. Do all of your shopping at one time, which will cut down the amount of time that you will put into thinking and preparing food. And keep it simple. The more you simplify planning and preparing meals, the less preparing and eating food consumes your life.

c. Take supplements. Bridge the nutritional gap that may be causing erratic cravings. (See my books, *Why Can't I Lose Weight?* and *Why Do I Need Whole Food Supplements?* listed at the end of this book for more information.)

3. Resist. *Submit yourself therefore to God. Resist the devil, and he will flee from you (*James 1:5-7). The devil tempts you with lies. Resist the devil's lies with the Word of God.

The battle over health and lifestyle is in the mind. The only way to deal with these unproductive thoughts is to recognize them and then choose to act on them.

We usually think it's our idea to overeat or eat the wrong foods. No, it's not necessarily. The devil wants us to think it's our idea. His assignment is to kill, steal and destroy (John

10:10.) One of his strategies is to get people to think wrong. He knows if we think wrong, we'll feel wrong and make wrong choices.

Have you ever felt bored, depressed or lonely and found yourself snacking on Doritos? We are vulnerable to the devil's subtle suggestions to make us feel better. Rather than recognizing this as a spiritual attack, we yield. We indulge. We eat the wrong food (Chocolate Sundae) at the wrong time. We feel good, and we forget our problem. We feel comforted. The problem is that we eat instead of dealing with the lie.

Your mouth has something to do with your ability to resist temptation. Watch what you say. Instead of saying, "I'm so weak," say, "I'm strong in the Lord." Your defense is the Word of God. Jesus spoke the Word, and He resisted the devil. You can, too! I recommend that you find scriptures that help you to overcome any bad habits.

4. Flee. Avoid temptations.

If you know you are tempted by donuts, then don't go to the bakery. Don't go to any where you are tempted for at least long enough so you can you break the pattern. If you are in the habit of going to the Git N Go or Quick Trip every morning for a cup of coffee and a donut, then stop the pattern. Don't go there. Plan to do something else. Don't go to the break room if it's a temptation for you. Stay away from vending machines. Use the God-given ability to form habits to your advantage. Break the pattern and replace it with a new one. If you don't do something long enough, it will eventually stop. If you do something new long enough, it will eventually take root. After a week or two, you will have broken the automatic pattern!

(For more help with changing your thoughts and behaviors, read my book, *Why Can't I Stay Motivated?*)

The word "mortify" means to gain control of physical desires by fasting (Romans 8:13.) God provided another great way for you to break these cycles through fasting. Let's go now to see how fasting helps us to "break the yoke of bondage."

Chapter Thirteen

God's Chosen Fast

When I was overweight, and struggling with some very bad eating habits, I used to wonder... how could I be so spiritual one moment and an absolute glutton the next—especially when bathing suit season was right around the corner?

In the Bible, Feasts honored spiritual remembrances, and special occasions. Most people know about Passover, or the feast which commemorates the flight of the Jews from Egypt. God gave the Israelites seven feasts to observe: Passover, Unleavened Bread, First Fruits, Pentecost, Trumpets, Atonement, and Tabernacles. Except for the Feast of Atonement, these feasts had special meals.

These feasts might encourage Believers that it's okay to eat a lot! Remember, there were only 7 major feasts, and their religious feasts were at the most a couple times a month. Think about modern day America. There is an excuse to feast nearly every month, and if you include birthdays and anniversaries, you could feast every week, or every day!

Overeating is hard on your digestive system. Earlier in this book, I discussed how processing foods makes us toxic. They create serious vitamin and mineral deficiencies and a toxic bloodstream. This is the beginning of every degenerative disease, including cancers.

The natural state of the body is divine health. Our cells are programmed for health and long life. So how can we keep them healthy? Through fasting.

First Corinthians 7:2 says, *Let us cleanse ourselves from all defilement of the flesh.*

Just as Jesus wants us to follow God's Health and Dietary Laws, He also wants us to follow His example of fasting.

Why Fast?

Fasting is a great way to break the cycle of addictions—to give up the excess sugars, carbohydrates or fats that are making us toxic. Fasting is God's way to cleanse both physically and spiritually. Fasting gives your body a well needed rest from digestion. When that happens, now your body can clean out the toxins, and allow natural healing processes which may have been hindered.

Physical Benefits of Fasting

There are many benefits to fasting. You will:

- Have more energy
- Cleanse your body
- Feel better about yourself
- Have a sense of victory
- Feel happier and healthier
- Retrain your taste buds
- Feel more motivated
- Normalize your metabolism
- Slow aging in your body
- Lower your cholesterol
- Get in touch with body
- Be more productive
- Have less cravings for junk food
- Purify your bloodstream
- Have more confidence
- Look better in your clothes
- Break the cycle of overeating
- Break your desire for sweets
- Improve your appearance/skin
- Help uncover food allergies
- Deal with stress better
- Lower your blood pressure
- Be able to break habits
- Control your weight easier

How to Fast

Rev. 22:2 says that the leaves of the tree were for healing. I started fasting with herbs more than 30 years ago. While Jesus fasted with water, today, most Americans are too toxic to water fast. I prefer a "semi-fast" purification program which allows people to cleanse while still maintaining normal blood-sugar levels. (The advantages of this fast is that it's easier, and while you don't have to fast entirely from food, you still can cleanse the body properly. You can learn more about it in my book, *Why Do I Feel So Lousy?*)

There are many excellent books on fasting, including *God's Chosen Fast* by Arthur Wallis, *Fasting and Eating for Health* by Joel Fuhrman, and *Toxic Relief* by Dr. Don Colbert which has several good chapters on fasting. While it's hard to give up all food permanently, most people can give up junk food. Whatever "fast" you choose, at least eliminate caffeine, sugar, dairy, meat and processed foods.

Beginning is the hardest part! It's so easy to keep putting it off. I get a notebook or just a pen and paper and I remind myself of my past experiences and victories. I remind myself of the incredible benefits of fasting and how great I felt during and after the fast. I remind myself of how much more time I had to spend with God; how much closer I felt to Him; how much easier it was to pray; and how much better I felt! If I have eaten too many snacks, or drank coffee, or even thought about food too much, I am reminded of how that all falls away when I fast.

Plan your fast. Write down your goal and put the dates on the calendar. Write down how you will fast, how long you will fast, and what you want from your fast.

You don't have to fast a long time to receive benefits from fasting. Even skipping a meal or two is beneficial.

Start with a twenty-four hour or one-day fast. That's reasonable for most people. In fact, some people are amazed at how easy it is. The first day might be hard, so you might choose a weekend so you can rest when you are tired. I prefer fasting while I work, because I'm so busy that I often forget to eat. Then you could move to a three-day fast. (That's just the 24 hour fast with two more days.) By the third day, most hunger pains are gone. I recommend you make an appointment with your doctor or natural healthcare professional if you want to attempt a fast longer than a week.

Watching TV may be hazardous to a fast. The advertisements are so superbly designed that they make you long for something to eat that you never knew you wanted!

Add Prayer

I want to encourage you to pray the Word of God. As you speak out the Word, it renews your mind. For example, pray that you love to eat good foods that God made for you; that junk food has no power over you; that it's easy to fast; that you love the way you feel when you fast; that you are loosed from the bonds of wickedness; that health vitality are yours; and that you can do all things through Christ who strengthens you.

Isaiah 58 is one of the most popular chapters on fasting. Verse 6 tells us what happens when people fast God's way: *To loose the bands of wickedness, and undo heavy burdens. To deal bread to the hungry and bring the poor that are cast out to thy house.*

Fasting is a great way to forget about yourself and minister to others. Let go of selfishness (ouch!). Then, after we have fed the poor and covered the naked, our health will spring forth speedily. Fasting like this is not a punishment, but rather a victory!

Spiritual Benefits of Fasting

Following a fast, you will:

- Increase your anointing
- Be more disciplined
- Enrich your prayer life
- Gain new perspective
- Be led by the Holy Spirit
- Overcome temptations
- Break bad habits
- Please God
- Break the cycle of sin
- Hear God's voice easier
- Have time to seek the Lord
- Be less distracted by the world
- Change your negative attitudes
- Consecrate yourself to God
- Be able to trust God more
- Increase your commitment to God

After the Fast

What you do after the fast will determine how effective the fast was! If you break your fast and just go back to old eating habits because you feel so much better, you will probably undo a lot of the good that you accomplished with fasting. Fasting is an important part of God's health plan.

My closing prayer is that you will slay any "Giants" of overeating or bad habits that you have been struggling with by following God's Dietary Laws and eating the foods that He designed for our bodies. May God richly bless your journey to health, and bless the works of your hands as you serve Him.

Endnotes

1. Roy Walford, *Beyond the 120-Year Diet* (NY, NY: Four Walls Eight Windows, 2000)

2. Don Colbert, M.D., *What Would Jesus Eat?* (Nashville, TN: Thomas Nelson, 2002), p.xi.

3. National Center for Health Statistics, 2000 "Leading Causes of Death" (Web address: www.cdc.gov/nchs/fastats/lcod.htm.)

4. World Health Organization Statistical Information (Web address: www.who.int/home-page)

5. Elmer Josephson, *God's Key to Health and Happiness* (Old Tappan, NJ: Fleming Revell Company, 1976), p. 25.

6. Carol Simontacchi, C.N., *Crazy Makers: How the Food Industry is Destroying Our Brains and Harming Our Children* (NY, NY: Penguin Putnam, Inc., 2000), p. 25.

7. Rick Weiss, "Correctly Prescribed Drugs Take Heavy Toll," *The Washington Post,* April 15, 1998.

8. Patrick Quillin, Ph.D., *Healing Secrets From the Bible* (N. Canton, OH: Leader Co., 1995), p. 16-17.

9. Jonathan Wright, *Dr. Wright's Guide to Healing With Nutrition* (New Canaan, CT: Keats Publishing, 1984), p. 4.

10. Nathaniel Altman, "Nutrition and Watergate: The Story of the Four Food Groups," *Health Quarterly,* April 1980, p. 72.

11. "Dietary Goals of the United States Select Committee on Nutrition & Human Needs," (Feb. 1977); United States Government Printing Office, Washington, D.C., p. 13.

12. Oldways Preservation & Exchange Trust 2000;

    (web address: www.oldwayspt.org/pyramids/med/p_med.html)

13. Paul A. Stitt, *Beating the Food Giants* (Manitowoc, WI, Natural Press, 1995), p. 117.

14. Paul Stitt, p. 117-118.

15. Paul Stitt, p. 121.

16. Lisa Messinger, *Why Should I Eat Better?* (Garden City Park, NY:Avery Publishers), 1993, p. 1.

17. Messinger, p. 3.

18. Sharon Broer, *Train Up a Child in the Way They Should Eat* (Lake Mary, FL: Siloam Press, 1999), pp. 38-39.

19. Sharon Broer, p. 38.

20. Marian Burros, "Additives in Advice on Food?" *New York Times,* Nov. 15, 1995, Vol. 145, p. C1.

21. Marian Burros, p. C1.

22. Dr. Norman Walker, *Pure and Simple Natural Weight Control* (Prescott, AZ, Norwalk Press, 1981), p. 51.

23. Walker, pp.51-52.

24. George Malkmus, *Why Christians Get Sick* (Shippensburg, PA: Treasure House, 1995), p. 42.

25. Simontacchi, pp. 4-5.

26. Simontacchi, p. 6.

27. Sally Fallon, *Nourishing Traditions:The Cookbook that Challenges Politically Correct Nutrition and the Diet Dictocrats* (Washington, D.C.: New Trends Publishing, Inc.,1999, 2001), p. 3.

28. Paul Stitt, pp. 246-247.

29. Carol Simontacchi, p. 42.

30. Carol Simontacchi, p. 50.

31. Barbara Stitt, *Food and Behavior* (Manitowoc, WI, Natural Press, 1997), p. 31.

32. Paul Stitt, p. 196.

33. Patrick Quillin, Ph.D., *Healing Secrets From the Bible* (N. Canton, OH: Leader Co., 1995), p. 16-17.

34. Mary June Parks, *Will Bible Foods Prevent Cancer?* (Frankfort, Kentucky: Parks Publishers, 2000), p. 21.

35. William Dufty, *Sugar Blues* (New York, New York: Warner Books, 1975)

36. Carol Simontacchi, p. 3.

37. Paul Bragg, *Healthful Eating Without Confusion* (Santa Barbara, CA: Health Science), pp. 14-15.

38. Nancy Appleton, Ph.D., Web address: www.nancyappleton.com.

39. Mary June Parks, pp. 22-23.

40. Barbara Stitt, p. 56.

41. Barbara Stitt, p. 47.

42. Bragg, p. 58.

43. Bragg, p. 59.

44. Don Colbert, *Walking in Divine Health* (Lake Mary, FL: Strang Communications, 1999), p. 30.

45. Dr. Royal Lee, "The Special Nutritional Qualities of Natural Foods," 1942, Report No. 4, pp. 38-39.

46. Dr. Royal Lee, p. 43.

47. Dr. Royal Lee, p. 41.

48. Paul Stitt, p. 126.

49. Paul Stitt, p. 140.

50. Paul Stitt, pp. 40-41.

51. *Nutrition Week*, March 22, 1991, 21:12:2-3.

52. George Malkmus, p. 44-45.

53. Dr. Reginald Cherry, M.D., *The Bible Cure* (Lake Mary, FL: Creation House, 1998), p. 8.

54. Sharon Broer, p. 173.

55. Mary June Parks, *Will Bible Foods Prevent Cancer?* (Frankfort, Kentucky: Parks Publishers, 2000), pp. 12-13.

56. Jean Carper, *Food—Your Miracle Medicine* (New York, NY: Harper Collins, 1993), p. 7.

Bibles Referenced

The Amplified Bible (AMP). Zondervan Publishing House, Grand Rapids, Michigan, 1965.

The King James Version. World Bible Publishers, Iowa Falls, Iowa.

The Message New Testament: The New Testament in Contemporary Language. Navpress, Colorado Springs, Colorado, 1993.

The New American Standard Bible (NAS). Life for Laymen, Denver, Colorado, 1977.

The New English Bible. Oxford University Press, October, 1963.

The New International Version (NIV). Zondervan Publishers, Grand Rapids, Michigan, 1973.

The New King James Version (NKJV). Thomas Nelson Publishers, Nashville, Tennessee, 1984.

The New Testament In Modern English, Revised Student Edition (Phillips). J. B. Phillips. Macmillan Publishing Company, New York, New York, 1972.

The Simple English Bible New Testament. International Bible Publishing Company, New York, New York, 1978.

The Way: An Illustrated Edition of The Living Bible as Developed by the editors of Campus Life Magazine, Youth for Christ International (TLB). Tyndale House Publishers, Wheaton, Illinois, 1971.

The New Testament in the Language of the People (Williams). Charles B. Williams. Holman Bible Publishers, Nashville, Tennessee, 1986.

The New Testament in Modern Speech (Weymouth). Kregel Publications, Grand Rapids, Michigan, 1978.

The Worrell New Testament (Worrell). Gospel Publishing House, Springfield, Missouri, 1980.

I have made every effort possible to check the accuracy of material quoted and obtain permission for any material or reference quoted beyond the fair use law. If there is any question, or a possible mistake in quoting of any material, necessary changes will be made in future printings.

Order Form

Please Print

Name _____

Address _____

City _____ State _____ Zip _____

Phone _____

E-mail _____

METHOD OF PAYMENT

Check _____ Credit Card: Visa_____ Mastercard_____

Card number _____ Exp. date_____

Authorization Signature _____

ITEM	QTY	PRICE
Why Can't I Lose Weight? ($17.95)		
Why Can't I Lose Weight Cookbook ($17.95)		
Why Can't I Stay Motivated? ($14.95)		
Why Am I So Grumpy, Dopey and Sleepy? ($11.95)		
Why Am I So Wacky? ($11.95)		
Why Eat Like Jesus Ate? ($11.95)		
Why Do I Need Whole Food Supplements? ($9.95)		
Why Do I Feel So Lousy? ($9.95)		
Subtotal		
Shipping & Handling Add 15%		
(Add 8% if resident of OK) Tax		
Total		

Send check or money order to:

Life Design Nutrition

Lorrie Medford, CN

PO Box 54007

Tulsa, OK 74155

918-664-4483

918-664-0300 (fax)

E-mail orders: lorrie@lifedesignnutrition.com

www.lifedesignnutrition.com